D1598004

WAKE · BAKE
&
MEDITATE

About the Author

Kerri Connor has been practicing her craft for over thirty years and has run an eclectic Pagan family group, the Gathering Grove, since 2003.

She is a frequent contributor to Llewellyn annuals and is the author of *Spells for Tough Times: Crafting Hope When Faced with Life's Thorniest Challenges, Ostara: Rituals, Recipes & Lore for the Spring Equinox, The Pocket Spell Creator: Magickal References at Your Fingertips, The Pocket Ritual Creator: Magickal References at Your Fingertips,* and *The Pocket Idiot's Guide to Potions.*

Kerri runs the Spiral Labyrinth, a mini spiritual retreat at her home in Ringwood, IL.

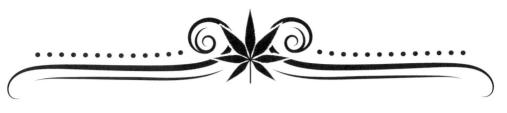

WAKE · BAKE

&

MEDITATE

Take *YOUR* **Spiritual Practice** *TO A*
Higher Level *WITH* **Cannabis**

KERRI CONNOR

Llewellyn Publications
Woodbury, Minnesota

FIRST EDITION
Second Printing, 2021

Book design by Samantha Penn
Cover design by Shira Atakpu
Editing by Annie Burdick

Llewellyn Publications is a registered trademark of Llewellyn Worldwide Ltd.

Library of Congress Cataloging-in-Publication Data
Names: Connor, Kerri, author.
Title: Wake, bake & meditate : take your spiritual practice to a higher
   level with cannabis / Kerri Connor.
Other titles: Wake, bake, and meditate
Description: First edition. | Woodbury, Minnesota : Llewellyn Worldwide,
   Ltd, 2020. | Includes bibliographical references.
Identifiers: LCCN 2020000485 (print) | LCCN 2020000486 (ebook) | ISBN
   9780738760636 (paperback) | ISBN 9780738760674 (ebook)
Subjects: LCSH: Hallucinogenic drugs and religious experience. | Cannabis.
   | Marijuana. | Meditation.
Classification: LCC BL65.D7 C67 2020 (print) | LCC BL65.D7 (ebook) | DDC
   204/.2—dc23
LC record available at https://lccn.loc.gov/2020000485
LC ebook record available at https://lccn.loc.gov/2020000486

Llewellyn Publications
A Division of Llewellyn Worldwide Ltd.
2143 Wooddale Drive
Woodbury, MN 55125-2989
www.llewellyn.com

Printed in the United States of America

Other Books by Kerri Connor

Ostara (Llewellyn Publications)

Spells for Tough Times (Llewellyn Publications)

*The Pocket Spell Creator: Magickal References
at Your Fingertips* (New Page Books)

*The Pocket Guide to Rituals: Magickal References
at Your Fingertips* (New Page Books)

The Pocket Idiot's Guide to Potions (Alpha Books)

Forthcoming Books by Kerri Connor

*420 Meditations: Enhance Your Spiritual
Practice with Cannabis* (Llewellyn Publications)

For Kahlen and River,
Your Ganja Grandmas love you

Contents

Disclaimer

Using, distributing, and/or selling cannabis is a federal crime and may also be illegal in your state or local vicinity. It is your responsibility to understand all laws pertaining to the possession or use of cannabis before choosing to obtain or use it. Neither the author nor publisher are accountable for consequences derived from the possession or use thereof.

Always seek the advice of a qualified health provider with questions regarding medical issues. This book is not a substitute for medical advice.

Acknowledgments

No book comes without help, so I have a few people to thank.

Thank you to:

Tammy for all the info on how to get my card—I should have done it sooner!

Tyler for being my coach.

Krystle for finding a Thursday babysitter so I could spend more time writing.

Taylor for being my first partner.

Brandee for helping with taste testing.

Mike for putting up with me and the weed smell.

Laura for everything, including taste testing and keeping me slightly sane.

BN 2959 for being the most supportive group of people I know. I love you and miss you all.

Everyone at Llewellyn Publications for allowing me the opportunity to make this book with you.

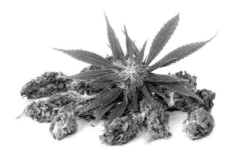

Introduction

Thank you for picking up this book. For whatever reason, it spoke to you. Whether you are interested in spirituality, meditation, or cannabis, something about this book spoke to you.

I would like to start by telling you what *Wake, Bake & Meditate* is NOT.

It is not meant to convince you to start using cannabis. It isn't here to tell you if you don't, you are missing out. It isn't intended to tell you to run out and break the law if you happen to live in a place where the smoking or consumption of certain plants is illegal. It won't tell you how to use different forms of cannabis or paraphernalia for consumption, but it will help you broaden your spiritual world once you do use them.

More specifically, it will teach you how to meditate with cannabis and will give you several meditations to practice on your own and with a group. Using cannabis to open your body-mind-spirit connection

to the divine is a deep and deeply personal experience. *Wake, Bake &*
Meditate will help you dive in. It will help you through your beginner
stages of learning how to use cannabis in a spiritual meditation, set
up your practice as a solitary, and then help you advance on to group
workings.

As a practicing Pagan, I understand there may be some debate
and concern about whether it is safe to use "mind-altering drugs" in a
practice. On that note, I would like to state the following.

In my opinion, cannabis is a plant. It is not a drug. It is classified
as a drug so that it can be controlled by the government. My hope is
that someday soon, maybe even by the time this book comes out, the
United States of America (as a country) will realize the value of cannabis and legalize. My own state has a medical compassion program and
just signed legislation measures to legalize recreational usage. Cannabis has been used as an entheogen for literally thousands of years and
has been illegal in the US for less than one hundred. History and facts
support the use of cannabis. Opinion and fear are its enemies.

You also do not need to be Pagan to use this book. It does include a
brief history of the use of cannabis in several different types of spiritual-
ism, showing how it has been used for centuries as a conduit to the universe and divine. Whatever your beliefs and practices are, you can easily
adjust the meditations to fit your own spiritual realm if necessary.

I do believe there are plenty of times when the use of cannabis is
preferable to unaided meditation, for several reasons. It can be a great
energy builder, a relaxant, an aphrodisiac, and, most importantly, a
channel to the divine. As a part of nature, it is indeed a gift from the
Great Creator, whomever you believe that to be. Using cannabis as a
part of a spiritual practice is not new, but in some circles it has been
frowned upon for generations.

After our dive into the history of spiritual use, we will discuss some basic cannabis information, along with recommendations of specific strains to use while meditating. Then we will go over experimenting, followed by the basics of meditation. When we finish those up, you will be ready to tie it all together to build and begin your practice.

The meditations in this book are progressive and should be done in order; each will be longer and more in-depth than the meditation before it. The individual meditations should be done first before you start on group work. Any of the meditations can be performed over and over again, but don't jump ahead in the lineup. Perform them in the order given. The order is designed to help you progress along your spiritual path. After you have completed all of them, you may go back and repeat any of them in any order you would like as the needs arise. Be sure you are getting everything out of the meditation that you can. Perfection is not expected; this is a *practice,* so feel free to practice all you need! You will also perform the meditations first without the aid of cannabis, and then again with it. It is amazing to see the differences in the same meditation once you add the boost from cannabis.

Finally, you will notice that I do not use the term *marijuana* in this book, and it's for a good reason. As Stephen Gray explains in *Cannabis and Spirituality: An Explorer's Guide to an Ancient Plant Spirit Ally*, the word *marijuana* was used by the first commissioner of the US Federal Bureau of Narcotics in the 1930s, Harry J. Anslinger. Anslinger led a racist attack against black Americans and Latino immigrants and their use of cannabis. Anslinger is largely responsible for the illegality of cannabis today, and if it wasn't for his views, many minority people sitting in jail today would not be there. The word *cannabis*, however, has been used in a positive manner for hundreds and hundreds of years (Gray 2017, 16).

In other words, just don't say marijuana; it's racist. We are starting to see changes in our society, with people realizing the inequality of enforcement and punishment regarding cannabis laws. As more states legalize, many are also starting to wipe out convictions and empty jails of people convicted of committing the "crime" of using a plant. While we still have a long way to go, progress is starting to be made. You can be a part of the solution by using your vote to change the legal status of cannabis and your voice to eliminate the stigma the powers that be have subjected it to for far too long.

When I first began using cannabis for pain, I had no idea the ways it would end up changing my life for the better and enhancing my own spirituality. It has helped open my eyes to my own faults in a noncritical manner and find solutions to problems. I hope you can find the same peace and happiness through your use.

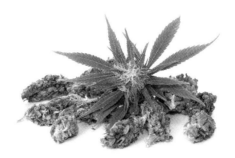

Chapter 1

Wake: A Brief History of the Spiritual Use of Cannabis

Cannabis has been around for thousands (according to some accounts, millions) of years, with humans partaking as early as twelve thousand years ago. Evidence shows use dating at least back to the Neolithic Age (Gray 2017, 2).

It has been used for generations by different religious groups all over the world. There are already several books on the market that go deeply into the sacred history of cannabis, so in this book we will only take a brief look. If you would like more information about the history of spiritual uses of cannabis, be sure to check out the bibliography and suggested reading at the end of this book.

While all these traditions are different, and each have their own beliefs and guidelines, one thing prevails throughout them all—the use of cannabis as an entheogen, a key to unlock and discover the divine within. It is a spiritual tool that has been used to connect mind, body, and spirit together in what Abraham Maslow named "peak experiences." These are described as mystical experiences in which one is able to transcend the self and feel at one with the universe (Ferrara 2016, 3). We will discuss peak experiences later.

Our journey begins in India, where the *Cannabis indica* plant is believed to have originated. Ferrara tells us cannabis was used in India before records were kept and structured religion was conceived, "a time when magic, mythology, healing, and sacrament blended seamlessly in shamanism" (Ferrara 2016, 13).

Think about this for a moment. Imagine a life where all these aspects are combined together in your own spiritual practice to heal yourself, others, and the world. This should be a part of our life's work. Our ancestors all over the world knew this, and it's time we remind ourselves and our societies of this again. While progress can be a beautiful thing, it's also the same progress that pulls us further away from each other, ourselves, and our spirituality. Imagine what the world would look like if everyone could feel the connection between healing and their spirituality.

The Vedic religion of the Indian region was known to use a soma beverage during ritualistic practices, named for the god Soma. Indian author Chandra Chakraberty explains in several books that soma is indeed cannabis, a view shared by many other Indian authors and researchers (Bennett 2017, 45). The *Rigveda* books contain many references to soma and its uses. This verse from Book 8 I find especially appealing: "We have drunk the Soma; we have become immortal; we have gone to the light; we have found the gods" (Ferrara 2016, 16).

Not only does this show the usage of Soma (cannabis), it describes its connection to deity. This complete feeling of peace, awareness, and connection far outweighs the damage any other humans can do to us. It overrides all negativity, hostility, and disapproval one may find in the outside world and instead fills us with confidence, awareness of ourselves and others, and a positivity we can carry with us always. This is healing from the inside out.

In post-Vedic Hinduism, Shiva became Lord of Bhang—another cannabis beverage that mythology tells us Shiva made from his own body. Dolf Hartsuiker, author of *Sadhus: India's Mystic Holy Men*, says the use of cannabis is a sacred act for self-realization and acquiring spiritual knowledge (Bennett 2017, 45–47). Someone who has hit a peak experience knows this to be true, but if you have not yet hit one, it may sound hard to believe. However, that is totally okay, because this book is going to help you get there to experience the oneness for yourself.

The Sādhus are holy people from the Hindu tradition who have given up worldly belongings and connections in the name of their spirituality. They are often seen dressed in bright yet simple orange or yellow gowns, with long beards and painted skin. Sādhus are well-known for partaking in cannabis, as they believe it will help them find "oblivion in the grace of God." Ferrara tells us that people in the Indian subcontinent (India, Pakistan, Bangladesh, Nepal, Bhutan, and Sri Lanka) used cannabis in religious practices and ayurvedic healthcare as far back as 1500 BCE, and saw it as a "food for the gods worthy of sacrificial offering" (Ferrara 2016, 29).

And while there appears to be no evidence that the Buddha used cannabis, there are several references suggesting he ate hemp seeds. The tantric sect of Buddhism (which holds far different beliefs than the main branch) was known to use the different parts of the cannabis plant for different reasons including as a "perfect medicine" (Bennett 2017, 48–49).

Moving on, the Zoroastrians of the Axial Age (from 600 BCE to the seventh century) in Iran drank a substance known as *haoma*—a combination of plant materials including cannabis and psychoactive mushrooms. This drink was designed to put the consumer into an altered state for a spiritual ritual. The Avesta scriptures (the sacred book for Zoroastrians) reference cannabis in different forms, such as the smokable bud and a potion (Ferrara 2016, 35). It was said to be used to "attain mystical visions that deeply influenced their cosmology" (Bennett 2017, 43).

As Islam rose and the Zoroastrians declined, some aspects were absorbed by Islam, particularly in the Persian Sufi sects. Muslims have a long history of sects on both sides of the cannabis question—while some prohibit it, others find it to be acceptable. The Sufis used it not only for the feelings it produced but for the creativity it unleashed (Ferrara 2016, 37–45).

This is one of my favorite aspects of cannabis—whenever my creativity needs a boost, it is remarkable how well it helps open my mind to new and evolving ideas. Honestly, I was high when I came up with the idea for this book, and for much of the time writing it. From William Shakespeare to Lady Gaga, weed has been used by many well-regarded individuals to boost creativity.

In Mithraism, cannabis played a small role in the spiritual workings of the initiates as they worked through stages to achieve the highest good. It was used in conjunction with breathing techniques, medicines, rites, amulets, and the repetition of magical words (Ferrara 2016, 36). Does the combination of these aspects into a practice remind you of anything? It's very similar to meditation, except many people today skip over including the substance that can open their minds the most.

We know *Cannabis indica* was being used in the Indian areas, but Kathleen Harrison also tells us cannabis seeds were used as food in China as far back as eight thousand years ago. They used a type of *Cannabis sativa* for food and for its fibers. Three thousand years later the Chinese used cannabis as a medicine, as offerings in rituals, and as an incense whose smoke could affect anyone who breathed it in (Harrison 2017, 23). Today, hemp is used for its fibers, food, and to produce CBD products. It's actively making a comeback, with more states legalizing hemp. The 2018 Farm Bill made hemp federally legal, opening the industry considerably.

As far back as the Neolithic (Stone) Age, Chinese shamans used cannabis as an important component in their rituals. Bennett reports that Chinese history expert Joseph Needham claimed both the Chinese and Taoists knew of the entheogenic properties of cannabis for thousands of years (Bennett 2017, 40).

According to Ferrara, the Chinese tome *Classic of Herbal Medicine* (authored by Shen Nong Bencaojing in approximately 100 BCE) tells us the prolonged use of cannabis allowed the user to communicate with Spirit and/or with ghosts (Ferrara 2016, 55). What the Chinese referred to as communicating with the "spirit light" is what we refer to as a peak experience.

Alchemically trained Daoists also used cannabis for entheogenic purposes and knew how to use it in different forms (such as smoked versus ingested) for different purposes (Ferrara 2016, 63). We can use the same knowledge to do this today.

The Greco-Roman Scythians also liked to get their bud on. Ferrara tells us of portable sweat lodges the Scythians used as early as the fifth century BCE to heal the spirit and mind, in which they would toss cannabis flowers onto hot stones to inhale the smoke (Ferrara 2016, 111).

I would only recommend adding intense heat (such as a sweat lodge or even a hot tub) once you are fully aware of how cannabis affects you and you have a bit of experience using it. Heat intensifies the effects of THC, so this isn't for beginners.

Recent discoveries have opened the door to more information on how the Egyptians used cannabis spiritually, medicinally, and recreationally. Testing of nine mummies revealed high concentrations of THC (Ferrara 2016, 73). There is some debate about whether the THC had accumulated through ritual and recreational use or if it was there due to medicinal use, since cannabis was also used as a sedative. Either way, to have results with high concentrations shows frequent use at least toward the end of life.

Even Christians from Egypt and Ethiopia smoked from exquisite ornate pipes to prepare for spiritual undertakings (Ferrara 2016, 77). There is something to be said for the device or tool you smoke from. I have many different pipes, along with concentrate vapes and dry herb vapes. Which one I use depends on the role I want the cannabis to play at the time. For my daily medicinal purposes, a vape or regular pipe is just fine. But when I am working spiritually, I have special pipes I enjoy using—my two favorites are one with a hamsa and one with an ohm symbol. I also have a rainbow-colored vape and a gold-colored vape to use in my practice.

The use of cannabis also spread alongside the spread of Islam, as the practitioners already knew what cannabis could do for them and they saw no reason to give it up. Its ability to increase perception levels was highly desired. Mystics who traveled from Syria to Egypt in the twelfth century brought cannabis with them and grew it as a crop. It was used in both spiritual and congenial settings due to its entheogenic and meditation qualities, and for being able to lower inhibitions (Ferrara 2016, 77).

Beginning in the sixteenth century, cannabis was used in the Sikh religion of the Punjab region. The Sikhs used bhang, a drink made with cannabis, in their religious practices to such a degree that its use is noted in the Granth Sikh scripture (Bennett 2017, 50).

In Nigeria, cannabis was used not only for peak experiences, but to communicate with the spirits of the dead. Its scent was used as an offering to entice the spirits to appear (Ferrara 2016, 78).

Many areas of Southern and Western Africa used, and still use, cannabis for fibers, textiles, medicine, and as an intoxicant. Zulu warriors used it before battle to eradicate fear, but they also used it as a medicine, for recreation, and to see the future (Ferrara 2016, 82).

According to Ferrara, African slaves who were shipped to Jamaica to work on sugarcane plantations brought their culture with them. Rastafarians rose from the slaves with a strong belief that cannabis was given to mankind for the "healing of the nations" (Revelation 22:2). In the Rastafarian tradition, the Tree of Life (as named in the King James Version), discussed in Revelation 22, is indeed cannabis. They cite Genesis 1:12 in support of their veneration of the holy herb: "And the earth brought forth grass, and herb yielding seed after his kind, and the tree yielding fruit, whose seed was in itself, and his kind: and God saw that it was good" (Genesis 1:12). Rastafarians use cannabis in many aspects of life, including food, medicine, tea, and ritual activities (Ferrara 2016, 95).

Each of these examples further confirms to us that cannabis has been used the world over for thousands of years to enhance spirituality in its many different aspects. While in some religions it has played a smaller, lesser role, in other religions it has been a necessity of spiritual practices. Today we can decide how much to incorporate cannabis into our own spirituality. We can also see that it is not the evil devil's weed some want us to believe it is, but merely a plant that has a long and expansive history of beneficial practice.

It is truly amazing the different views cultures can have on something as simple as a plant. While some cultures have found uses medically, emotionally, and spiritually, others have vilified the plant and labeled it as evil. I must assume that was due in part to people who feared the power of cannabis, especially in a spiritual sense. What would it mean for modern-day structured religions if all you needed was the aid of a plant to feel at one with the creator? Combine that with its medical capabilities and it becomes easy to see why big pharmaceutical companies and others in health-related fields might want to vilify cannabis and keep it out of the hands of the people. It's taken close to a hundred years here in the United States, but at least we are starting to fight back and reclaim the legality of cannabis.

I will admit, when I first began medicating, I felt like I was doing something wrong, something bad. I felt guilty because I had been raised to believe the lies that cannabis could kill you. My nine-year-old mind saw a *Quincy M.E.* episode called "No Way to Treat a Flower," and though the weed the victim smoked and died from in the episode was tainted with poison, that part was glossed over in my house. It was emphasized that weed killed the girl. Once I became interested, it was more than illuminating to find that cannabis has been used for thousands of years as an incredibly effective medicine. Basically, you could say that getting doped made me realize that I, and millions of my fellow countrymen, had been duped. Cannabis was not the evil danger society had led us to believe. I went from feeling like a hypocrite to feeling anger about having been lied to, especially about something that could have been helping me for decades while instead I spent years on medications that could have killed me. That anger has now been directed into educating others, bringing cannabis back into our lives to be used as needed, and most importantly, allowing individuals to have the choice to use it if they wish.

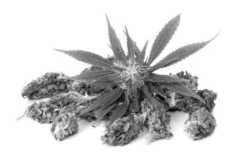

Chapter 2

Recommended Strains
for Spiritual Use

The next thing we need to explore are the different types of cannabis. I was never aware of the different types before I began using
cannabis, and now that I do know, I have found people who have been
using it for decades and still don't know much about the different types
and strains either. Seldom did people in the past have any idea what
strain they were getting (and many street market buyers still don't);
it was just "weed." But now there are many unique strains, with more
being bred all the time. These new strains are being created for special-
ized purposes—for example, higher THC or CBD content.

Cannabis is first divided into three main categories: sativa, indica,
and hybrid.

Sativa plants are tall, thin, and have skinny leaves. They have a higher THC to CBD ratio, which energizes and relieves fatigue for the user. Sativa plants are uplifting, alleviate depression, and improve attitude. These strains are more apt for daytime use and generally would not work well with most (but not all) meditations. Some meditations— particularly for group work—benefit from the energy building of sativa that can then be released into the universe. These strains are excellent for trance dancing to high energy drumming. A sativa (or sativa-dominant hybrid) with a high THC and lower CBD ratio works best for high-energy meditations.

Indica plants are believed to have originated in the Hindu Kush region near Afghanistan. These plants are short, stocky, and have a thick coat of resin that protects the plant against a harsh environment. Indica strains have sedative effects that aid in improving sleep, stimulating the appetite, and relieving pain. The sedative, couch-lock effects allow your body and mind to relax; these strains are therefore a good fit for connecting with the divine and for other spiritual uses.

The last type of plant is a hybrid between sativa and indica. One strain will be more dominant in each hybrid, depending on who its "mother" was, as the female strain is always the dominant one. Hybrids can be used for a variety of purposes, including relieving anxiety, inflammation, and insomnia. Hybrids can also be used in many different meditative states, depending on the meditation and the dominant strain. Hybrids are created to "weed" out some of the negative effects (I know, bad pun), while emphasizing positive ones. They are also created to help provide relief for different medical ailments.

THC and CBD are two of the cannabinoids found in the cannabis plant. THC is primarily what gives cannabis its psychoactive effects. CBD works in a tranquilizing manner, which means the higher the combination of the two, the greater "high" you are likely to experience.

CBD can also counteract some of the more negative effects of TCH, such as anxiety or paranoia.

Due to legalities, it may be difficult to find certain strains in certain areas. At this point, anyway, it's not like we can just go online and legally buy whatever strain we want. For this reason, I am including several different strain options, so you can find what is more available to you in your area. You should also try to use a variety of strains throughout your practice. Your body will become too accustomed to the same strain if you use it over and over and don't vary it. This makes achieving a high and peak experience more difficult. Find at least a few strains that work for you and shuffle their use around.

While different strains can produce different effects, the most common negative side effects are dry or "cotton" mouth, dry or itchy eyes, anxiety, and paranoia. The key to avoiding anxiety and paranoia has to do with your dosing and tolerance level. We will discuss more about dosing in later chapters. The other side effects can be dealt with by keeping plenty of water on hand, along with a bottle of eye drops.

Recommended Strains

Because you will want to use indica strains for most of your meditations, I will start with these first. Indica strains usually cause the munchies, so I'd advise you to keep a simple snack on hand. If you need to maintain a high, you can also use the recipes at the end of the book. If you are doing shorter meditations for which maintaining a high or peak for an extended period is not necessary, your choices are open. I prefer bite-size fruit, berries, grapes, or chunks of watermelon. Not only do these satisfy the munchies, but they help with cotton mouth issues and provide extra hydration.

Indicas

These indica strains will produce the following positive reactions: relaxation, sleepiness, happiness, euphoria, and uplifted mood.

Granddaddy Purple (Gdp)

The very popular Granddaddy Purple or Purps has a distinct taste and aroma that I personally like. A cross between Purple Urkle and Big Bud, it does have a bit of a grape/berry flavor to it, making it lighter and not as earthy or dank as some strains. It is a very common strain and has a high availability. It's in my top five favorites for reliability. I prefer to use Granddaddy Purple in more uplifting meditations rather than deeper-thought, transcendence type of meditations, as it tends to give me the giggles—a side effect I only find in a few strains.

Kosher Kush (Kos) and Hindu Kush (Hk)

Hindu Kush and Kosher Kush are very similar to me, without many differences, except for taste and scent. These are two strains I can always fall back on if Northern Lights isn't available. A light dose of either of these puts me in a good, happy, uplifted mood. It does take me a much larger dose to hit a peak with these than with Northern Lights, but again this is only my experience; you may find the exact opposite to be true! Like Northern Lights, I prefer to use both Hindu and Kosher Kush for deeper, more focused meditations of a transcendant nature. If it has "Kush" in the name, I am game.

Lavender (Lar)

I have only been able to find this a few times at my local dispensary, but I really love it. I like to describe it as "velvety smooth." It does have a hint of lavender to it. I like this strain very much and have had great experience with it, but unfortunately it isn't available to me very often, and with its cost, "stocking up" isn't always an option. It gives a light-hearted, giggly high and is better suited to uplifting meditations. It is the perfect accompaniment for Midsummer meditations.

Northern Lights (Nl)

Northern Lights is my favorite, and most of the time it is my first choice for spiritual meditations. If it's available when I head into my dispensary, chances are I will pick up at least an eighth or a vape cartridge to make sure I always have some on hand. The first time I hit a peak experience was with Northern Lights. Whether I use flower, oil, or a resin vape, I can always expect to have a good journey with this strain. While I used to get slight cotton mouth from it, it was bearable, and as my body got used to it, the dry mouth has gone away. I find this strain to be the best for me when it comes to spiritual journeys, and I highly recommend giving it a shot to see if it works for you. I prefer to use Northern Lights for more focused, deep meditations.

Sativas

Sativa strains produce the positive effects of creativity, physical and mental energy, euphoria, and happiness. You won't hit the same kind of peak with sativa as you do with indica, but you will experience an uplifted, energetic clarity. These strains are perfect for trance dance or other more physical activities or meditations, such as drumming.

Sadly, most of the sativa strains that are most recommended in many articles related to meditation are not available in my state, so I have never been able to try those! This is one of the big issues with not being able to buy over state lines. California is able to get Lamb's Bread, Laughing Buddha, and Malawi Gold—the three most highly recommended strains for meditation, according to other authors and websites—but here in Illinois, I have not been able to try them. Laughing Buddha and Lamb's Bread are at the very top of my list if (hopefully when) they become available in my area. Ultimately, this means I had to do a lot of trial and error testing of sativa strains to find which would work best for me and are popular enough to be found in many locations.

Clementine (Clm)

Clementine is the child of Tangie and Lemon Skunk, which gives it a great citrusy taste and smell. I prefer the vape to the flower in this strain, to eliminate the smoke, giving it a "cleaner" feel. The taste and scent of the vape is literally almost like candy. This gives me a bit of the buzzed feeling throughout my body, while keeping my head clear and focused. I find this perfect for trance dancing, as the energy and focus are present while my body can enjoy the movements for the physical pleasure it produces. This is my favorite sativa strain.

Durban Poison (Dp)

Durban Poison was the first sativa I ever tried. It took some getting used to after consuming only indica for several years. It's a sweet-smelling bud, and with this one I prefer flower over vape or concentrates. It gives plenty of energy and stamina with a good level of focus. Its use is ideal for drumming or faster trance dance meditations.

Sour Joker (Soj)

Sour Joker was the second sativa I ever tried, and I still go back to it on occasion to keep it in my rotation. It gives you a buzzed head high with a well-defined area of focus. For me, Sour Joker creates a bit more of a relaxed than energetic feel, so I prefer to use this for slower physical workings—spiritual dance meditations that are more flowy in nature but require stamina.

Tangie (Tg)

If you can't find Clementine, there is a good chance it's mother, Tangie, may be close by. Tangie was created in Amsterdam from California Orange and Skunk #1. It is a pretty popular and more readily available citrusy breed that is very similar to its offspring Clementine. With Tangie I find the same positive effects, but I can't get quite the depth of feeling as I do with Clementine. It's a close second for me, as it also offers a great citrusy taste and scent, and again I prefer this in a vape too, for that "cleaner" effect.

Hybrids

Hybrids are the result of pairing sativas and indicas together, the mother plant being the dominant one. By combining plants, geneticists can "weed" out certain traits and side effects and emphasize others. These combinations can increase or decrease THC, CBD, or other cannabinoid counts, along with terpenes. Cannabis research has made such strides in just a few years; the possibilities of what can eventually be created are limitless.

Alien Rock Candy (Arc): Indica Dominant

Alien Rock Candy is my second favorite strain. I have had some of my best experiences with Alien Rock Candy, although I also had my worst experience with it too, which was my own fault for not going "slow and low." I had first used Alien Rock Candy in a vape. Generally, a vape hits people harder and faster than flower does. Generally. For some reason, I did not have that experience the first time I smoked an Alien Rock Candy bud. I smoked a bowl and it hit me far harder than the equivalent of what I would have vaped. My paranoia (not a common side effect with this strain) was sky high. I woke up my husband and made him stay awake with me until the feeling wore off. Since then, I have learned to take it much slower, particularly when trying something new or in a different form. This is another reason why it is beneficial to be able to have THC, THC-A, and CBD count information, and actually use it. Having the information doesn't do any good if you don't pay attention to it. (Obviously, I'm guilty of messing up a time or two, but again, it's a practice—no perfection required.)

Alien Rock Candy provides a deep concentration that allows me to easily hit a peak out-of-body experience.

Blue Dream (Bd): Sativa Dominant

Blue Dream is an interesting strain, as it tends to invite in creativity and mental stimulation but not deeper intense concentration, while at the same time providing an uplifting, euphoric feeling. I often find it to be the perfect combination from both sides. For meditation usage, I like this for happy, upbeat group meditations. Plus I love the name!

Bubble Gum (Bg): Indica Dominant

Bubble Gum is a high-THC hybrid that is well-balanced with a fruity taste. Vapes will give you a purer bubblegum taste than flower will. It gives a great heady high and feeling of euphoria, with a boost of creativity and a body buzz. This strain is also for happy, upbeat meditations.

707 Headband (707): Indica Dominant

This hybrid is another with a high THC level (which personally I prefer in my hybrids). This strain gives a creative, heady high. A cross between Sour Diesel, OG Kush, and Master Kush, it has been used to treat anxiety, making this an excellent strain for those who are prone to anxiety or paranoia side effects. This one is best for upbeat meditations that also take place in a relaxed environment.

You can probably tell from some of their effects how different strains affect certain types of meditations. Obviously, if you are working on a highly serious meditation, a strain that tends to make people giggly would not be appropriate. But for a more fun, lively meditation, it might be just what you need.

The side effects are also something you need to pay close attention to. While dry mouth can easily be combatted by having hydration close at hand, paranoia is more difficult to deal with, particularly in a group meditation.

Therefore, it is extremely important to know how a strain works with your body chemistry. Different people react to different strains in unique ways. You need to experiment with strains and dosages to find what works best for you.

Even when participating in a group meditation, you may need to use your own individually chosen strain, as others may have a completely different reaction than you do. We will discuss this more in the next chapter.

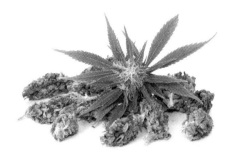

Chapter 3
Bake: Time to Experiment

This is my favorite chapter in this book because this is the chapter in which you get to learn all about being yourself and discovering what works best for you. While experienced users might already know what their dosage requirements are, we are also going to cover setting up the different aspects of a meditation practice. We won't just be covering weed in this chapter—we will be exploring several different types of experimentation to set you on your path, headed in the right direction.

While some of you probably already consume cannabis and some of you probably already meditate, this chapter is going to take care of the prep work to combine these two activities together in an organized manner that will help you physically, mentally, emotionally, and spiritually get into the practice.

Before you get into the basics of experimenting with cannabis, you need to start by preparing your tools and setting. Let's begin with what will become a very important part of your practice, especially during the experimentation process: your journal.

Journal

The journal you use for this practice will be very personal to you. It will contain not only your usage information, but your deeply personnel revelations, feelings, thoughts, and emotions. Whom, if anyone, you choose to share your journal with is up to you. If you do build into a group practice someday, imagine the intimacy you will experience if you and your group members do decide to share your journals with one another. Cannabis use invites intimacy into your life in a truly uninhibited manner. Where you decide to take that is up to you as an individual practitioner of course, but in a group setting, intimacy itself breaks down barriers, allowing for closer, stronger bonds that result in stronger, more powerful magic and workings.

Your journal will, in a way, serve as a Book of Shadows. It should be treated with reverence and honor. Therefore, be sure to show it the respect it deserves. In other words, don't pick up a notebook from the local discount store. Make this journal something special. I personally love either hand-bound books or leather-covered books, or combinations of the two. I have seen leather-covered binders that allow for the removal and replacement of pages. Whatever works for you and creates a feeling of respect when you look upon it and work with it is the one you should use. You may go through several journals over the course of your practice, but this one will always be your first. This one will document those first moments of intention toward hitting your peak experience. This one will always document the first steps on your journey, and it may indeed be something that you one day feel the need to share with others, perhaps as a partner helping someone on their journey.

Your journal entries should be kept in a chronological order, with each entry dated. Be sure to include information regarding the strain used, THC count, THC-A count, CBD count (if this information is available to you), method of consumption, dosage, and time of consumption. This is all your technical information. (We will discuss this more when we get to dosing.)

Begin your journal by writing out a dedication to your practice. You may want to use something like "I dedicate this journal to the spiritual journey I now embark upon with cannabis as my guide."

Next, set an affirmation for your practice. Include this in your journal and before each meditation. I use "I grow with each step I take. I learn with each breath. I will bloom and flourish along the way."

Questions to Write About

Consider these questions and then explore them in the pages of your journal.

1. Why do you want to undertake this practice? What are your expectations?

2. Describe the area in which you will perform your meditations. How does it look now? How will you change it or add to it to make it your perfect meditation location?

3. Do you need to purchase or find anything to complete your area? If so, write out your shopping list.

4. What do you like best about your meditation area?

Setting

The other information you will want to include is what is called "set and setting."

Your "set" is what you bring into your experience. This includes your beliefs, emotions, and intentions. Your "setting" is the environment in which your experience takes place (Gray 2017, 17).

For our purposes, we want to create the most spiritual set and setting we can. This poses the question of where your sessions will take place. You will need to make sure it is a location in which you will be able to both comfortably meditate and comfortably consume in your chosen manner.

Over the summer, I had a bell tent set up in the yard (until the humidity just got to be too much). This was no ordinary tent, though. It had a circular gray rug, dozens of large meditation pillows, and a memory foam twelve-inch-thick mattress. The bedding and pillows were done in a bohemian pattern of pink, orange, teal, purple, black, and white. It was my haven for a while, and where parts of this book were conceived and written. I was able to smoke without bothering anyone and I could meditate and contemplate and work without anyone bothering me. The breeze and sounds of wind chimes and nature from my two-and-a-half acre wooded yard were precisely what I needed. Unfortunately, we had a particularly wet and hot summer and I needed to pack things up before the humidity did permanent damage. I hope someday to replace the tent with a yurt or cabin instead.

You obviously do not have to go to the extreme of a yurt, or even a tent, but you can if you want! What matters most is that the place you choose is comfortable for you. When you first begin, you will be using a partner, so the ideal location must be able to provide comfort for the both of you, but it does not have to be the ideal location for both of you. You each get to decide what works best for you as an individual.

You also don't always have to practice in the same location. If you can practice outside, by all means do it! Invest in some decent meditation cushions you can carry to your location. (Just be aware of laws regarding the consumption of cannabis. Don't get caught consuming somewhere that isn't legal, or even just being somewhere that isn't legal). Part of my property is wooded, and I look forward to practicing outdoors in the fall, with the cooler air and the beautiful foliage, often with a small firepit nearby. This would always be my most ideal location, but unfortunately fall only happens for a few weeks out of the year here.

My indoor meditation is done in my yoga/meditation/infrared sauna room. This is my indoor haven. I have different options for my meditation positioning, including several meditation pillows, a "Rama Meditation" chair, a zero-gravity chair, the sauna itself, or just a yoga mat with conveniently placed bolsters. As someone with fibromyalgia, rheumatoid arthritis, and ankylosing spondylitis, my comfort needs vary by day, so it is important for me to have these different options to help deal with any physical flare-ups.

You need to make sure you do what you need to make the space comfortable for you. If the space works for both you and your partner, that is great, but if it doesn't that is okay too. You won't be "taking turns" in the same session. Some people prefer to be indoors, while others only like to meditate outside. I'm lucky enough that I have a place for meditation both indoors and out. Depending on where you live and your living arrangements, you may be confined to one or the other.

If you have land, find a spot that calls out to you. You will want something in the shade, so you don't have sun glaring into your eyes (even if they are closed, it can be hard to concentrate when it's bright) and to prevent sunburn. Tall grasses can help hide you from the world and the world from you. Maybe you have a flower garden that will work. Whatever is most comfortable for you will be the best option. Try out different spots in the yard. Take a moment and just sit with your eyes closed. Is the grass too scratchy? Will you need a blanket? Is there a rock poking your hind end? Do what you must to make your location perfect.

If you need to be indoors, then you need to follow pretty much the same steps. Make sure you aren't in a location where the sun will shine right in your face through a window. Make sure it's going to give you peace, quiet, and privacy. You want a place that calls calmness, serenity, and tranquility to mind. If you have the space for it, design your own meditation room. Bring in whatever you need to make it comfortable for you: a heater, fan, blankets, pillows. Make this your sanctuary. What do you need to be comfortable? Some people prefer the minimalist approach and like a yoga mat with maybe a neck roll and bolster. Others may prefer the snuggly sinking comfort of a pillow pile. Use your creativity to create a space that is sacred for you. This space needs to require a bit of effort in planning; that doesn't mean it has to be elaborate, but again, don't just throw something together. This is the place you want to be when you experience a closeness with Spirit and a oneness with the universe. Make it reflect that.

While designing your space, you will want to take into consideration your seating and lighting arrangements. Some people are more comfortable meditating while seated, others while lying down—just don't get so comfortable that you end up constantly falling asleep. With the added relaxation of some good ganja, you may end up falling asleep several times in the beginning. It will be up to you and your partner to decide how you want to deal with situations like that, which we will discuss more in a bit.

If you can meditate outside, you will want to sit on the ground as much as possible. You may need to put a blanket or pillow underneath you for comfort, but don't use a chair if you can help it. If you really do need a chair (trust me, I know how hard getting to and from the ground can be!), try using a zero-gravity chair. Remember your partner can help you with it if necessary. A zero-gravity chair in a reclined position helps keep your body in alignment with the earth. It can also add to the lightweight floating sensation of a high. Otherwise, keep yourself as connected with the earth as possible. Lie down outside if you want, but you will probably need at least a thin pillow under your head, and perhaps a sheet beneath you. Bolsters can help add to outdoor comfort, or even to your indoor setup. If you want a pillow pile outside, then do that. Try a hammock. Whatever it takes to bring you peace and focus in a safe, comfortable location.

When it comes to lighting, there obviously isn't much you can do about it outside during the day, but if you meditate at night, you may want a lighting source. Candles may not work well outside, depending on the type of candle and how breezy it is, but you can always try lanterns or torches for a glowing fire illumination.

If firelight is not an option, try flashlights with either different colored plastic lenses or different colored lightbulbs. Blue is a very calming color and may help soothe you into your meditation. Color-changing, LED, battery-operated touch lights are easy to transport and can be used for brightness during setup and then tapped into a different color mode to create your desired meditation atmosphere.

Inside you can use just about any type of lighting you want: candles, colored lights, salt or crystal lamps, even lava lamps. All of these can help you set a mood that is peaceful and relaxing, yet still gives you enough light to see so you don't fall over something while trying to get up or run into a wall trying to find a light switch. Some people do prefer to meditate in complete darkness, but this may not only be a little unsafe, it may also make you fall asleep. Try a blue or violet lighting arrangement to calm yourself, but also to give you enough light to keep things safe. No matter what you use, your lighting should be soft, not glaring.

There are other items, such as statues, plaques, crystals, and gemstones, that you can add to your room or space to help enhance the mood for the meditation you are about to undertake. You may want to change these mood enhancers to correspond more with the meditation you are performing. Nothing is set in stone. You can make these changes whenever you want. Experiment to find out what works best for you.

Music is a key factor to help you get into a meditative state of mind. There are a ton of songs designed specifically for meditations and yoga. Look for albums that have natural music—these are songs with sounds from nature mixed in with the music. I personally love Sequoia Records and Paradise Music.

Some meditations work better with certain types of music, while others work better with other kinds of music. This is going to be up to your own personal taste, but I do recommend building as large a meditation music library as you can, just to give yourself more options. When you listen to a song, think about what it means to you and what the music is saying to you, and then find a meditation that ties in with those same thoughts. You will find perfect combinations this way. Use sites like Pandora or Spotify to help discover new artists and songs.

Candles are good for more than just your lighting. They help set the mood for your meditation. Blue and white candles have calming effects and may help you sink into your meditation more deeply.

Purple and white also have spiritual qualities. You may also want to choose colors that correspond in some way to the meditation you are going to perform. (*Llewellyn's Complete Book of Correspondences* by Sandra Kynes is a great reference tool to keep on hand.)

Candles also come in different scents and you may find something that really helps you relax, but also provides light and ambience at the same time. Otherwise, you can burn incense or drip a few drops of essential oil onto a lit charcoal tablet (in a fire-safe container) to release a strong burst of scent into the air. Lavender, frankincense, and patchouli are all meditation favorites, but you will want to experiment with different scents to see what works best for you. Look into the correspondences of different scents to find one that will reinforce the purpose of your meditation. My favorite go-to prepackaged incense is Ganesha from HEM Incense. This scent has been extremely helpful to me in learning to meditate, and since I use it so often, my brain now associates the scent with meditation, providing me with an excellent trigger that helps me slip into a meditative state.

Finally, you can bring in decorations to help enhance your meditation. Pictures or statues of your deities are always a nice addition, along with other representations of nature such as plants, flowers, crystals, or a small water fountain.

Even if you can't set aside a designated space that is only used for your meditations, find a space you can use and then bring in what you can to make it more special during your sessions. Pack those items up at the end of your session and keep them safe in a nice box or chest. Again, choose something that shows these items are honored for their purpose and the role they play in your spiritual meditative sessions.

As you begin the meditations or as you begin your dosage experimentation, you may find that what you thought would work simply doesn't, and you may have to make some changes. This is all an experimental process for finding what works for you and what doesn't. Trial and error are a part of any practice. Simply use what you learn to make your practice better, more comfortable, more complete, and closer to your peak every day.

Dosing

Now that you have your location set up, let's talk about dosing.

The information available to you will define what kind of specific dosage details you have. I can walk into my dispensary and purchase strains in packaging that contains specific information about their THC and CBD levels. This is information that isn't available to most small personal growers if they have no methods for testing. That being said, it doesn't mean you can't still learn how to dose yourself accurately—even if you don't know precisely what the dose is.

First, I want to cover cannabis that has analyzed cannabinoid levels. There is also a big misconception I want to cover here. Just because someone uses medical cannabis does not mean they have ever hit a peak experience, or even been high at all. I am in an online medical cannabis support group and asked my fellow group members (a very active group of fifteen thousand people) about their peak experiences and was surprised to see how many knew very little of the spiritual uses of cannabis at all; few had actually achieved their own peak experience. For medical users, the rule of the road is slow and low. Low doses slowly until you learn your tolerance level and where you feel the best. For many, many medical cannabis users, this is as far as they go. They use it to help their conditions and to relieve their pain, not to get high. I can't tell you how many medical patients I have spoken with who not only haven't been high, but are scared to even try. This is a big reason why I highly encourage the use of a partner when you are starting out. It's awesome to have someone there to reassure you throughout the process. It also builds an extreme intimacy because you will find yourself being very open and uninhibited with them. This can be a scary prospect for some people, but the cannabis also helps you face that fear. (More on this when we get to partnering.)

If you know the percentage of cannabinoids and what doses are necessary to help your symptoms without getting high, you know your starting point. That is where you will start your slow and low process from. For example, if you normally vape two hits of a 30 percent THC indica for pain relief, start with three inhalations and go from there. Give your body and mind time to react to the new dose to see how it feels.

It's important to remember while doing this that different forms of consumption need different amounts of time to take effect. Edibles take longer to have an effect but provide a longer sustained high. This can also vary greatly from person to person. This shows the versatility of the plant itself, as it can and does affect people differently. A strain that might work well for me may make a friend of mine nauseous. The same goes with dosages. The most important lesson of this chapter is that everyone is different, and everyone will be affected somewhat differently. You must learn what works well for you.

If I am looking to hit peak quickly for a short working, either smoking or vaping works best for me. However, if I need to sustain the experience, then I use a combination beginning with an edible, followed by smoking flower, and add a vape when/if necessary for a boost. This is what you will want to aspire to eventually: to know your body and the effects of THC on it well enough that you know what it is you need to hit different levels of "high."

If you have access to those analysis numbers, this is one way you can keep track of what your journey will require for a successful round trip. Most of the time. I say most of the time because some people do build up a tolerance level depending on how often they use cannabis. This problem can be solved in a few different ways.

First, prevention. Don't overuse to begin with, then you don't have to worry about building up a tolerance in the first place. This option is pretty much not in the realm of possibility for medical users, as many of us already deal with tolerance issues and medicate daily out of necessity, not for a high.

Second, rotate strains. Pick out a few different strains that work well for you. Mix them up. Try using each one for only a few days at a time before moving on to a different but similar strain. This has helped me, medically, from getting overly tolerant to one strain and building a resistance to it. It helps with this type of use too.

Three, take a tolerance break. It's that simple. Don't use anything for a week or two. Give your body a chance to eliminate some of the THC built up in it. While everyone has their own "remedy" for removing THC from their system, the most efficient manner is … don't consume any new THC and let your body work it through. Time—that's all it really takes. You also don't have to wait for every trace to be gone; you only have to lower your levels enough that a normal dose again has the same effect it once did.

More important than knowing the actual percentages of THC you are consuming is noticing how it feels to you. If you are new to consuming cannabis and are going to smoke flower, you need to make sure you learn how it affects your body and mind every step of the way. This is more of the experimenting you get to do. And you get to do it over and over again before you even combine it with a meditation.

As I've stated before, when it comes to dosing, you are going to start low and progress slowly. You also are going to pay very close attention to how each dose makes you feel. For smoking, it's generally recommended to wait up to twenty minutes in between doses to feel the full effects. That's all we are going to be concerned with for a while—feeling the full effects of each dose, documenting them, and learning about how cannabis tends to make you feel.

While seasoned users have felt a high or already elicited peak responses from the pipe, virgin users can find the task intimidating. There is a good reason why I want you to ease into a high if you haven't before, or even if you have, but you've had a bad experience in the past and are approaching the act with some trepidation. Cannabis, particularly certain indica blends, can definitely trigger anxiety. If you are already anxious, it can increase that anxiety. While some hybrids do help decrease the chances of anxiety caused by use, beginning your experience already anxious may not give you the best experience. On the other hand, the cannabis may relieve your anxiety! This again all goes back to the importance of going low and slow and documenting along the way.

This is an entirely different way of learning how to get high than what many people have experienced in their lives, the biggest difference really being the intention behind the high. My very first time getting high as a teenager had literally nothing to do with anything spiritual. It was done more to find out what the big fuss was about and to get friends of mine off my back about trying it out. Simple peer pressure. All through high school I had friends that used, but I never did. I was always the clean, sober one who made sure everyone got home safe and sound. I wasn't a partier, though I went to parties. I wasn't just a designated driver, I was THE designated driver. So over winter break my senior year, when I finally decided to give in at a party one night, my friends were a bit surprised. Turned out they would also be a bit regretful. After smoking a bowl, with no real set intention whatsoever, I hid my head under a blanket, with my friends laughing at me, until the munchies hit. We went to a local restaurant where I consumed a large Greek salad. I followed that with a piece of triple chocolate cake. After the cake, I decided I was hungry and ate another entire large Greek salad. Followed again by a piece of triple chocolate cake. After three salads and three slices of cake, my friends dragged me out of the restaurant and swore they never wanted to be around me high again. I didn't get high again for another year. It would take many more years before I actually learned about getting high and setting an intention along with it. So, if you have been getting high for years, but never with a set intention, don't feel bad! We can work on changing that and opening you to a new world of focus, clarity, peace, intention, Spirit, and, of course, magic.

While you are experimenting with different doses, your biggest tasks are to be aware and to communicate what you experience to your partner. Your partner's job will be to assist you in maintaining your comfort and your high (when necessary), and to document your feelings, statements, reactions, and so on. Some people may want to film or audio record their sessions, and while this is entirely up to you, I don't recommend it for several reasons. For one, there is the possibility of legal issues depending on where you live. No need to give anyone unnecessary ammunition. Second, people watching themselves on any type of video is often uncomfortable. You may not like what you see, and this may leave you with another wall to bring down. Third, being filmed may leave you feeling somewhat vulnerable, therefore not being able to fully let go and give in to the high. Fourth (yes, I have a few reasons!), it's impersonal. This is an intimate journey between you and Spirit, being documented by your partner. Keep it sacred. The less technology involved the better. While you may need technology for things like lighting and sound, let's draw the line there.

Because cannabis is different for everyone, you must know yourself to know what you need and what works best for you. I cannot emphasize this enough. The only way to get to know what works best for you is to experiment and find out.

At the end of the chapter we will go over specific exercises on dosage experimentation, along with how a session should be recorded. Right now, let's take a little break from reading and answer a few more journal questions.

Journaling Questions

1. What is your "set"? What are your views on and experiences with using cannabis? How were you raised to view cannabis? How have your views changed now? Are you just beginning to use? Medical patient? Long-term consumer? Are you nervous? Are you excited to begin your journey?

   Take some time to really think about your answers. Try to be as specific as you can be about what you think and feel about the experience at this time. It will be interesting to look back on in the months and years to come.

2. If you are a regular or experienced user, tell the story of how you came to use and when. What were the views of society about cannabis at that time? If you are new, what brought you to this point in your life?

3. If you are a regular user, what is your normal consumption on a weekly/daily basis?

Partners

Even if you are an experienced user, I highly encourage you to use the partner system. I have met and known "stoners" my entire life who have quite literally spent decades high, and many of those people have not used cannabis as a spiritual tool or to connect with others or with Spirit. In fact, many of them use it as a form of escape, but don't make the full journey to escape from the body but still connect with the mind. To those who have used for spiritual and connection purposes, you may still want to use the partner system; your input would be invaluable to a beginner. Partners do not have to be teachers, but should be able to feel comfortable in a supportive role. The issues that need support in each partnership can vary greatly. If one person has experience with consumption and the other with meditation, obviously they can work to help each other out. But you may be in a situation in which neither of you has consumed or meditated, or both have done one, but not the other. You may even find yourself wanting to work with different partners somewhere down the line to see what you can learn from and teach each other. For now, you will need to find a partner you want to work with to begin your journey.

Your partner is your confidant. You will want to make a lot of considerations before you choose your partner. While your partner does not have to be someone who wants to use cannabis for meditation, they do need to be 100 percent supportive of YOU using it. If you cannot find a truly equal partner—one for whom you can perform the same tasks as they do for you—then a nonuser is the second best option. And who knows, maybe learning from your experiences will change their mind and make them decide it is something they would like to pursue further.

Our culture has demonized cannabis for so long that it is difficult to totally throw aside the lies and propaganda and the stigma that has gone along with it. More and more people are opening their eyes and their minds to the possibilities of cannabis, though, so your experiences may have a positive influence on others. You may also find that some of the people you might like for your partner are stuck in a situation where they want to overcome fear but would rather watch someone else take those first steps. If you are comfortable with a situation like that, by all means, go ahead. But also remember that the intimacy you experience, the oneness you experience, will not fully be comprehensible to your partner. They will not experience what you experience, so they also won't be capable of true understanding.

What other qualities should your partner have? They must be trustworthy to you. They must be aware. They must be committed—learning dosages can take a while, and you don't want someone who isn't going to have the patience to stand by you and wait. They should be discreet—I'm going to assume you don't want someone who is going to be blabbing your business all over Facebook. Your partner may be a spouse, significant other, close friend, coven or other group member, or maybe just someone else who wants to experiment too. The important aspect is you must have trust with this person. If you are in a position where the only people who are supportive of this practice are people you don't know that well, spend some time getting to know them! In today's world, we want everything right now, now, now. In the word of cannabis, "now" has an entirely different feeling to it, which you will soon realize. Relationships and spiritual practices both take time to build, and it's time well invested to bring about peace of mind to the practitioner. Build relationships with people who are supportive of your journey.

They must be able to understand that they need to not only pay attention to what you say and tell them, but to observe your nonverbal actions. They must be able to provide comfort in the case of anxiety issues, nausea, or a bout of depression. These are the things people who have not gotten high tend to worry about. Your partner is there to assuage your fears, to provide support and comfort, and to document everything. Let your partner know what you will want and need from them. You may need a bit of coaxing to discuss your feelings; let your partner ask you questions as you go to help increase communication and the flow of information. If there is a problem—perhaps you feel nauseous—they should stay on top of it and make sure the feeling has passed. As you get deeper into the high, your inhibition may drop, making it easier to convey your feelings, but the higher you get, you might also need to be reminded that you actually need to open your mouth and speak in order for your partner to hear you. While you may feel this incredible connection to the universe, your partner won't be able to read your mind!

Don't let any of this scare you; the documentation and awareness aren't because something bad may happen. It's simply so you can learn about yourself in relation to cannabis use so that you can have peaceful, stress-free, meaningful meditations. Once you learn about yourself, your needs, and your limits, you can fully experience and enjoy the benefits this plant has to offer.

While some reading this may think, "Geesh lady, lighten up, we don't need partners, we just need to smoke," please realize that with the introduction of legal medical cannabis to some states, there are a LOT of people who have literally never used before. With more and more states having recreational legalization, there will be even more people willing to try. I know it may seem very fun and easy for many people, but there are also many people who have been brought up to believe weed is simply evil and will hurt you or make you do crazy things, and even though that stigma is being attacked from all sides, it can still be a scary experience for some people. For those who are seasoned users, it's your job to help others who are interested in seeking out the benefits of this wonderful plant.

Session One

How far and how long you decide to go in each session is going to be completely up to you, but for this first session, I recommend setting a good two hours aside to "work," with time afterward for "recovery."

Decide with your partner what course of action you would like them to take if you fall asleep—in other words, do they let you sleep it off, let you have a bit of a nap, or wake you up? This is a personal decision and up to you. What you do today you don't have to do the next time either. For your first session, you may want to just sleep it off, but again, completely up to you.

To prepare for your session you will need:

- Your partner
- Cannabis and whatever equipment you need to use it
- Your journal
- A notebook for your partner
- Writing utensils
- Drinking water
- A small bowl with coffee grounds or lemon zest OR a bottle of lemon essential oil
- Your prepared location (including proper lighting, seating, music, blankets, pillows—whatever you need to be comfortable)

Turn your music on and relax. You may want to perform some quick and easy breathing techniques such as slow and deeply held breaths, or even do a few yoga postures, such as child's pose or *sha-vasana*. Use the affirmation you wrote in your journal. If you use my earlier example, that would be *I grow with each step I take. I learn with each breath. I will bloom and flourish along the way.*

This can easily be turned into a slow hypnotic chant or song to help focus your mind to a spiritual working.

Remember earlier I mentioned set and setting? The location you have prepared is your setting, the "set" is your mindset. Cannabis simply works best when you allow it to work. Sounds easy enough, doesn't it? But it isn't always. I still often find my mind fighting against me when I'm trying to get to sleep at night. Being an insomniac for decades, it can be very difficult for me to quiet my mind enough at night to allow the cannabis to do its job. If you fight the effects, they won't be the same as if you allow them to happen. Kick back in your setting, relax, and try your best to focus your mind on how you are feeling. This will also help block out other thoughts. For new users, this can be very difficult. I learned not to fight it in a rather bizarre way, one that had far more to do with my dentist than consuming cannabis.

Have you ever had nitrous oxide (aka laughing gas)? Being one of those people who freak out at the dentist, nitrous oxide is my friend, but it wasn't the first few times I used it. My natural instinct was to fight the effects of the gas, as I felt like I was suffocating. I wasn't, of course; it was panic, and I was doing it to myself. Once I learned to let the gas work and to "sink" into it, I found my dentist trips to be much easier to deal with. The first few times I used cannabis at all, I had no idea what I was doing. Sure, I had a little buzz, but I definitely had no clue how to enjoy it. When I began using it for pain relief, there was still so much anxiety—I was in massive pain and literally didn't know if I was going to live or die. I was highly paranoid that the doctors must know more than what they were telling me, because they were telling me they knew nothing about the infection I had somehow contracted. I was paranoid at even having cannabis in my home. I was scared half to death of what people would think if they found out. (And now I'm sitting here writing a book about it!) I was stressed to my limits. It took a while for me to allow the cannabis to ease my nerves along with easing my pain. It took even longer to be able to allow myself to enjoy it and then explore the possibilities.

When you are ready, go ahead and begin your dosing. Your partner (or you) will have written down the time, dosage, method of consumption, strain information, and whatever other details you have available to you to record. Your partner can use just a regular notebook to record your session, and as you review the notes, you can transfer them to your journal and make any edits or additions as necessary.

If you are an old pro or a medical user, you already have an idea of what it is going to take to get you high, but I want you to follow along with this exercise and still have your partner record your observations. Chances are you probably haven't focused this much on the process before, and it is interesting to go back later to see what patterns your usage may form, and to really focus in on what you feel and what you experience. You aren't just getting high for the fun of it, you are getting high to make a spiritual connection. How this plays out is partially dependent on how your body responds.

After each dose, allow some time for it to work. Mentally scan your body. What do you feel? Speak out loud so your partner can record your thoughts.

If you are using something like a vape, the effects can be almost instantaneous. I have seen several people who are occasional to frequent flower smokers be very surprised to see how fast a vape could hit them. Not to mention, the percentages on vapes are increasing all the time. When I began writing this book, 30 percent THC was the norm here in Illinois for medical vapes. Now, just a few months later, 70–80 percent THC is available from the same companies. Until just recently, I generally found flower to work faster for me, but now because some of the vape oils are so high in THC, I have a quicker reaction to them. Again, each person is different and so are the effects.

Seasoned users may not need as much time between doses. Just be sure you are fully exploring and communicating exactly how your body and mind feel. New users, feel free to take your time. It's not a race. After taking a dose, exploring, and communicating, go ahead and take your second dose. Your partner will record the time of each dose.

At some point, there are several different common side effects you may feel. Some are positive, some not so much, but be sure to convey these to your partner. You may find a pattern in how you experience them. These common side effects include a case of the giggles, a smile that won't quit, sexual arousal, the feeling of pins and needles or a light electrical flow through your body, forgetfulness, cotton mouth, nausea, and munchies. These side effects will also vary depending on the strain you use.

When you are ready for a third dose, go ahead. In this first session you are not looking to hit a peak experience, just a decent high. You can go further in your next session. For a new user, it may take quite a few sessions before hitting a peak experience.

You may be wondering why I said to have some lemon zest or oil or coffee grounds on hand. In case you feel like you have taken too much, the terpenes in lemon and coffee may help "bring you down" when you inhale their scent. Experiment with this a little to see if it works for you. Terpenes are the oils in the plants that give the strains their different scents and flavors. In some states, working with terpenes has become very popular and they are able to use terpenes extracted directly from the cannabis in cooking. In other states, like where I live, this is still a dream.

New users may be completely good in their first session with just two or three doses. This should be enough to get a high going for a newer or never-before user. Vaping, again, may take even less. While there are many different ways to use cannabis, some, such as dabbing, are more complex and should be left to those with more experience.

This first session is a mere introduction to cannabis itself and the overall process of setting up your location and working with a partner.

Journal Exercise

When your session is complete and you are ready, take some time to record the thoughts and feelings you have now about the process, what it was like, what you remember. Do this before you read your partner's notes, so you can compare your own recollections to what was previously documented. This is important not only to see what you remember, but to see how well you are communicating to your partner, and how well they are receiving your message. Include anything from your partner's notes, such as dosage information and any other notes they made. Your first time is over. If you were nervous, write about how you feel now that it's over. Was it anything like what you expected? What sensations did your body experience? What thoughts came to mind? Document everything you can.

Subsequent Sessions and Peak Experiences

Some people are only going to need a few sessions to hit a peak experience, while others may take several. Feel free to move at your own pace, but still commit to pushing yourself a little further along in each session. If you find you have any problems arise, use your next session to try to work around those issues. Commit different sessions to different strains until you find yourself comfortable with a few different variet-ies and confident about how you will react to them.

Again, new users may want to take a slower road that includes sev-eral sessions before going for a peak experience, while others may feel ready sooner—either is fine as long as you are comfortable with what you are doing.

Before working toward a peak experience, spend some time sim-ply enjoying the high. Give yourself several sessions of this. You can always come back to this at other times when you need to unwind and relax, so learn now how to get yourself into that "happy place." Know what it does for your body and the joy it brings your soul.

Once you have given yourself a chance to simply enjoy the high, it's time to learn how to use it to expand your awareness and mindfulness.

Dussault tells us in *Ganja Yoga* that "energy flows where awareness goes. If you pay attention to the high, you'll amplify it, creating an even more open, expansive state of awareness" (Dussault 2017, 63).

Pay close attention to your senses. For me, the first noticeable sign of hitting a peak experience is how suddenly my hearing seems to be far better than normal. Normally, it kind of sucks and I often find myself asking my husband to turn up the TV. Not when I'm really high!

In the summer, sitting out on my deck at night is one of my favorite times to hit a peak experience. My skin begins to tingle all over as I can feel my hearing kick into high gear. The sounds of my backyard at night are just incredible. It would be about impossible for me to not feel the close connection to nature that I do on those nights. Crickets, frogs, owls, bats, and other critters of the night create a symphony of music with their calls to one another. Being out in a rural area, the main light sources are the moon and stars, so it can get pretty dark. However, it also offers a spectacular view of those stars, and shooting stars can be seen with an abundance I had not known was possible before moving to my current home. It is one of the few ways I am able to relax and feel completely at peace, at least on a temporary basis, until my peak experience wears off.

Once you learn how to be aware and mindful in your high, you will then be able to push through the final barrier to hit your peak experience. When you realize that your awareness and mindfulness have connected you to Spirit, you have hit the peak.

While it may feel different to different people, one thing that all peaks do have in common is the feeling of the spiritual awareness of your surroundings.

When I am indoors, I need my background music to help take me to a peak. For me, my meditative state is extremely dependent upon what I am hearing. It is far more difficult for me to meditate or hit a peak experience without *sound.* Some people need silence to meditate, so this too is going to be something you need to experiment with to see what works best for you. Even the volume can help or hinder your journey, so do keep that in mind. I have a very specific level of music I prefer—not too loud as to be overly distracting, but loud enough that I can feel myself get lost in the sound. I also use music to help me sleep at night, but that is at a lower volume, so even though I medicate before bed, generally in high doses, the music is far more "white noise" and not at the level I like to get lost in when hitting a peak experience. Very similar dosing to what I would use for a peak experience, but the music helps anchor me and focus my energy into going to sleep instead. As an insomniac, it really does take me focusing on sleep to actually get there. It is very difficult to describe to people who either don't have that problem or are the exact opposite—narcoleptic and can't stay awake. Cannabis has helped me add an average of three hours of sleep a night to my life. However, because the dosing for a peak experience and sleep are so similar for me, it's easy to see why you need to experiment a bit to see what works for you. I kept falling asleep when trying to meditate, until I turned the sound on my music up and discovered the difference that made for me.

I realized this when I was outside one night meditating under the stars. I was astounded by how loud it seemed out in my backyard. I even thought maybe it just seemed that loud because I was stoned and I knew how it helped me fine-tune my hearing. So I pulled out my phone and just started recording in the dark. Turns out it *was* loud—it wasn't just me. I figured if it being so loud outside worked out well for me, I would try turning up the volume a bit inside, which of course ended up with positive results.

I hear people say all the time that they can't meditate, they can't quiet their mind, but meditation isn't necessarily all about quieting the mind. It's about focusing the mind, and cannabis helps even those of us who often feel like a complete scatterbrain to tone things down, once we learn how to use it most effectively for our needs.

Meditating does not come easy for many people, but cannabis can and does provide a magical boost to help you on your path.

When you do first hit a peak experience, you will know. You may have an overwhelming sense of awareness, of joy. You may feel that all things are connected to one another, yourself included. The feeling of true oneness with the universe. You may cry tears of gratitude and love. You may simply sit in awe. You may do all of these things at the same time, or one after another. But you will know.

I go through a particular pattern; it may vary slightly from time to time, but for the most part it follows this order:

1. Hearing intensifies

2. Warm, electric flush starts at the top of my head and flows down my body all the way to my toes

3. Massive power surge and intensified heat in the chakras

4. Cotton mouth

5. Nausea

6. Spinning

7. Sinking (This sinking is sudden, like a drop landing. I land in my sacred space.)

8. Floating in my sacred space

9. Another massive power surge in the chakras, followed by white spinning light in all of them. As this happens, I am able to send my energy out all around me, to share and blend with anyone I invite in. Their energy is then able to be shared and blended with mine.

Some of these things aren't fun; however, the cotton mouth and nausea do not always happen. Even if they do, they are a signal for me to push through to the peak that is coming. Yes, I have hurled a few times. You might too, but once your body gets more used to it, this will happen less often. Often these negative side effects happen to me for one of two reasons. It may be that I am using a new strain that I'm not as used to. The other reason is that I'm not allowing myself to let go enough. I have to remind myself to follow cannabis into the high and beyond and not try to lead it. Cannabis guides you to your sacred space and then allows you to take over. Fighting it will often induce negative side effects. If hitting a peak was easy, everyone would already be doing it. It's not easy, but don't let that scare you off. Anything worth having is worth working for. Once you are able to hit your own peak, you will quickly realize the effort was worth it.

There are also documented benefits to hitting peak experiences. According to Ferrara,

> researchers at John Hopkins found that all participants in whom peak-experiences were elicited, including novices and experienced meditators, gained a heightened sense of personal well-being generally accompanied by altruistic feelings toward others, greater aesthetic appreciation, increased sensitivity and creative thinking, and a broad-minded tolerance of others' viewpoints and values… As should be evident from the investigation the milder and gentler cannabis plant offers access to many of the therapeutic benefits of stronger entheogens, and most notably when combined with concentrated activities (such as meditation, contemplative prayer, chanting, or other such exercise) to actualize self-transcendence (Ferrara 2016, 105).

Imagine living in a world where this was the norm instead of what we have today. We can make the world like this, even if only in our own circles. It's up to us.

We have covered quite a bit in this chapter, so now I'm going to turn you loose for a bit. Your assignment is to do another twelve sessions with your partner. Each time, be sure to record your dosing information and your reactions. By pushing yourself a little further each time, you should be able to hit a peak experience at least a couple of times within your twelve sessions. Be sure to document everything about it. Do they feel the same to you each time? What differences are there? How do they make you feel? These experiences will probably feel miraculous to you, and that is just the beginning. Next, we are going to work on some meditation basics, and then finally we will get to combine the two practices together.

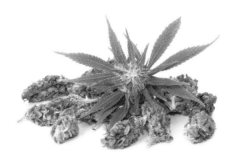

Chapter 4

Meditate: Bringing the Mind into the Mix

If you don't already have a meditation practice, this chapter is an important one for you! You need to first learn to meditate on your own before adding cannabis to the mix. This chapter will teach you the basics of meditation.

What Is Meditation?

Generally speaking, meditation is the practice, skill, and art of shutting all thoughts out of your mind other than those you wish to concentrate on.

It can be soaring through a cloudless sky, swimming in a crystal blue pool, walking through a lush green forest, or going places you've never been. It can help organize the thoughts in your mind. It can help you heal yourself emotionally, mentally, and physically, along with helping you de-stress after a hectic day. It is intentional mindfulness and awareness. It is expanding your conscious to meet your subconscious and communicating with the divine.

Meditation can be different things for different people; it all depends on the purpose behind your meditation. Some people will meditate for only one reason, while others meditate for many different reasons. What meditation is to you is for you to decide.

The tools and skills you learn to use here will help you begin a lifetime practice of meditation.

Tools for Meditation

When we talk about tools used for meditations, we are talking about actual physical items that will help you relax and perform your meditations. Skills are the mental and emotional "tools" you will learn to help you on this journey.

We will be working with visualization and guided meditations throughout this book. When you are first learning a guided meditation, you obviously won't have memorized the words to it, and trying to read while performing a meditation is counterproductive. Memorization also may throw you off, as you will be trying too hard to remember the exact words, so your focus will be on the wrong thing. Here you will learn how to get around those problems.

First you will need to find music that helps you relax—something calming and soothing, and preferably without any lyrics. When you have lyrics, you may tend to start singing along instead of focusing on the meditation at hand. When first starting out, you will want to give yourself more time to relax and get into the right frame of mind. Your "pre-meditation" music should last about two to five minutes. Don't go too long either, or you may end up boring yourself and giving your mind too much time to wander. You will need to experiment to find what works best for you.

Next you will also want "background" music to go along with your meditation. This may be the same music you used for your pre-meditation, repeated a few times, or it may be something else entirely.

Finally, you will need to record yourself reading the meditation out loud. Once you have your pre-meditation music recorded, turn your background music on and record yourself reading the meditation script as the music plays. Be sure to read through the script several times first to familiarize yourself with not only the words themselves, but with the timing and feeling of the meditation. Do not speak too fast. Take your time. Leave pauses when you feel they will be necessary. Once you finish recording the script, allow the music to play a little bit longer to give yourself time to slowly come out of the meditation.

As you become more skilled in focusing your mind, you may want to eliminate some of the pre-meditation music. After performing the same meditation several times, you may feel you don't need to be guided anymore and simply use the background music alone instead.

Invest in some decent headphones to help block out any other sounds. Even if you are performing a meditation indoors, you may want to use headphones. These will block out ringing phones and barking dogs.

You can also use your partner in this respect too, by having them read and guide you through the meditation. While a partner isn't 100 percent necessary to start your meditation practice, you can begin your journey together through these beginning sessions if you wish. If you want to be able to cover more ground without having to worry about scheduling sessions with each other, know that this part is something you can do on your own by using a simple recording device as described above.

Once again, you will be using your journal to help you focus your actions, thoughts, and intentions first on paper, then you'll transition this focus over to your mind.

Getting things sorted out on paper, where you can physically see it, makes it much easier to be able to see those same things in the mind's eye instead. You will also record your meditation observations in your journal after each of your sessions.

Skills for Meditation

As I stated earlier, many people do not believe they have the skills necessary to meditate. We all have the skills, we just need to practice using them. I do believe it is probably more difficult for people to meditate today than it would have been thirty or more years ago. Our world has changed so much through little shifts over the past thirty years with the electronics and smartphone age. Thirty years ago, to be online required a lot of heavy computer equipment, a landline, and some decent computer knowledge. In other words, our electronic distractions have sped life up in a way that has made us constantly "busy" without being *busy*. We experience constant, almost nonstop stimulation. We do not relax in the same ways we used to. This can make it seem very difficult to focus on one thing, but what this really means is that it can seem very difficult to focus on *certain* things when we tend to hyper-focus on several things at once, like TV, video games, social media, and cell phones.

We need to reclaim our skills of relaxation, focus, and intention to be able to put forth our best meditations.

How do you normally relax? Do you turn on the TV at night and veg out? Do you read a book? While these can both be relaxing to a point, they still require outward stimulation. Your body may be relaxing, but your mind is not. Society teaches us that we must be stimulated all the time, but that doesn't give our minds much of a chance at conscious peace. Start spending some time in simple, quiet relaxation. Turn off the TV, put the book down. If you absolutely feel the need for sound, play soft instrumental music at a very low volume. Spend time with yourself, just being. Don't think about what happened at work or school or the grocery store. Just breathe and allow your body and mind to take a break.

Focus is also a skill we must learn to adapt to the situation at hand. In this case we must learn to change our focus from outside stimulation to inside stimulation. We must focus internally to work through our first several meditations. I believe you will find that the way these meditations are designed, they will truly help you learn to focus inward when needed. We live in a society today that appears to be afraid of inner focus, and it hasn't been helping us. We need to look inside to learn and fix what we can in order to make our world a better place.

Intention is one of the greatest aspects of magic, and cannabis use. Coincidence? I don't think so. Our intention is our most powerful magic and it is our intention that gives cannabis its power. If we want to get high and be happy, cannabis obliges. If we want to be deep and introspective, cannabis obliges. Our will dictates where cannabis will guide us, but we must make the commitment to follow it.

Starting Your Practice

Time to stop talking about it and get started. When it comes to meditating, practice and experience will be your best teachers.

First go back to the area you chose to use to practice your dosing. Do you have everything you need to meditate comfortably? Your area should be set, but comfort is going to be even more important right now. Since you won't be using cannabis just yet, you may need to make adjustments to provide the most relaxation and peacefulness you can obtain.

In your journal, write out what your intention is. In these first several sessions, we will be working with deep breathing and visualizations to aid in relaxation. Finding a relaxing peace is the goal.

Get yourself situated for deep belly breathing. Place your hand on your stomach and inhale deeply through your nose, allowing your belly to push your hand out. As you exhale, feel your hand slightly press on your belly, and allow the air to escape through your mouth with a "wooosh" sound. Let it all out. Do this a few times with your normal breathing pattern, and then slow it down a bit. Count to three as you inhale, hold for three, and then again count to three as you exhale. Focus on the air coming into and going out of your body. Visualize the air as a white light, a beam of energy that comes into your lungs and your belly, and branches off into veins with its brightness cleansing everything in its path. When you exhale, the dim, grayer "exhaust" is dispelled in the opposite motion, exiting through the mouth.

As you feel yourself calm and relax, go ahead and slow your breathing down even more by increasing your count to four. Give yourself several inhalations and exhalations at the four count, and then slow your breathing down a touch more by increasing the count to five. Continue to breathe at this pace for several minutes. If you have music playing, allow yourself a full song of this deep relaxation breathing, along with the visualization of the cleansing white light.

When you are done, take a moment to check in with your body and see how you feel.

Journal Exercises

1. How did your body and mind respond to this deep breathing exercise? Could you visualize the white light? Did your body feel more relaxed?

2. What issues did you have with breathing and relaxing, if any?

If you were not able to feel the difference, spend the next few days trying this exercise again. When you are able to feel your body relax and can visualize the light, spend the next several sessions repeating this exercise, but while increasing the breath counts. Do a few days to a count of six, then seven, then eight, and so on. Only go until your comfort zone is stretched, but not gone completely. You don't want to be gasping for air, but you are training your lungs to breathe in a way that they are not used to. While I know plenty of people who can do this exercise at a ten count, I certainly have never been able to do it successfully. I also have asthma, so an eight count is where I am the most at ease. Again, this will take some experimentation to find out what works best for you. As you work on lengthening the count you use, also work on lengthening the amount of time you spend doing this breathing meditation. Add a little time each day until you are comfortable and capable of spending fifteen minutes doing this meditation. Set a timer or use music as your judge of time passing.

Always remember to use your journal beforehand to set your intention. After each session, write about how it felt. What do you notice about your body and mind while doing these exercises? What are you focusing on? Do you find your mind drifting off toward other things? It is important to document your thoughts and feelings on the exercises as they are performed now, so later you can look back and compare your reactions to doing the same exercises with the aid of cannabis. It also helps get you into the habit of using your journal, which helps focus your attention. When you go through the same steps each time you practice, you are creating your own ritual.

By the time you have found your comfort zone with your breathing count, you will have a bit of experience creating intention, focusing, and visualizing. Taking this slower, ritualistic approach to meditation by first learning to focus and meditate on your own breath may make it easier for you to overcome some of the hurdles you may believe you'll have with meditating. Setting up this ritual trains both your mind and your body.

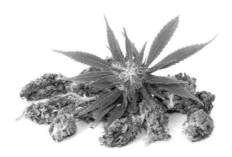

Chapter 5
Your Solitary Practice

Creating your own practice requires just that—practice. While it's okay to skip around a bit with your scheduling while you are in the experimenting phase, it's also okay to set aside a specific time even in the beginning to get yourself into the habit of a weekly practice. Once you have the basics down, it's time to get serious, so if you haven't set a specific day and time, do so now. If you and your partner can meet weekly, that is perfect, but even if you can get together only once a month, make the commitment and do it.

You will perform each meditation several times first without cannabis and then with cannabis. You do not want to use cannabis right away with any meditation, because you will never have the chance to fully see it again at the more basic level. Being able to progress slowly through the meditations allows you more time to fully explore your thoughts and your feelings, and will give you a better base to compare your meditation to when you do it again with cannabis. Practicing the meditation on its own without cannabis a few times also helps you to learn the meditation so that it is easier to progress through once you are aided by cannabis. Using cannabis will open your mind's eye to new and exciting thoughts, feelings, and ideas. Once you have experienced those aspects of cannabis use with each distinct meditation, you will bring something new to it each time you perform it, making it impossible to see it *without* the new information ever again. Ideally, I recommend performing the meditations in the following pattern: three times without cannabis then three times with cannabis.

How you do this is entirely up to you and dependent on how much time you have available; the beginning meditations are shorter and would be possible to do several times in one session. But you may also take your time and spread them out over weeks. Remember: you don't have to have your partner present for unaided meditation sessions. You can work on your "regular" meditations during the week, and then when you meet up with your partner, work on them with cannabis. How you decide to work on these meditations is up to you, and it all depends on what your prior experience with meditation is. If you already have a meditation practice, this will be a breeze for you. If you are just starting out, at least try the meditation by yourself (unaided) to see how you do. It might not be as hard as you think. The most important aspects of these meditations are to compare your unaided with your aided reactions, so you can see what the difference is like for yourself. Your journaling should be completed each time you perform the meditation. Follow that by reviewing your journaling from the previous session, and then you can document and discuss any new details you discovered.

The meditations we do will be progressive in nature. They will start off short and simple and grow in both duration and complexity. We already started with a great breathing exercise and we will move on to some easy visualizations to begin with. A visualization is simply a meditation that allows you to use your imagination in a limitless manner.

The individual meditations we will work on will also be centered around one typical theme: you. These meditations are for inner workings. They are ways to learn about yourself, to open yourself up to new people and experiences, to heal past wounds, and to discover who you are. When we move on to working with a group, those meditations will focus on outer workings—on our outer selves, how we see ourselves in our environments, how we can change the world for the better.

Meditations for Your Solitary Practice

Each meditation we do is going to be set up into the following sessions: sessions one, two, and three without cannabis and sessions four, five, and six with cannabis.

How many sessions you complete at a time is up to you. All meditations are going to begin the same way, with the "pre-meditation" provided below. This will be the beginning of each meditation we do, so you can refer to it as needed.

These meditations do need to be worked in the given order, as they do build upon each other. At any time, you can go back and repeat previous meditations, but do not skip ahead.

This chapter is your guide to your practice and will include step-by-step instructions in the beginning. As you progress through the meditations, you won't have to be told the same things over and over, as many of the steps will become habit and second nature. This is another reason it is important to follow the meditations as planned; skipping around would be counterproductive to establishing your meditation ritual. Repetition trains your body and mind, so we will use it as a tool. Eventually, you will be prompted to reevaluate how things are going and make any adjustments needed at that time.

The first few meditations are simple to follow and are not written in a script format. You should be able to read through them a couple of times and then perform them. However, if you are more comfortable in a guided situation, they can easily be scripted.

In many of these meditations we work with a higher power such as a deity or guide, but let your own belief system be your overall guide. If you do not work with higher powers, focus on something you do work with—your breath, energy, chakras, or nature. Make it about what works for you.

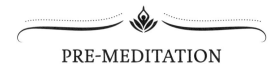

PRE-MEDITATION

Set your mood. Turn on your music, light your incense and candles if you're using them. Document the time. (When we get to working with cannabis, document dosage information. If you want to create sacred space or a protective circle, do that now.)

Write down your intention in your journal. (This will vary depending on which meditation you are doing.)

Get yourself situated in a comfortable position for your meditation. We will begin with deep belly breathing. Place your hand on your stomach and inhale deeply through your nose, allowing your belly to push your hand out. As you exhale, feel your hand slightly press on your belly and allow the air to escape through your mouth with a "wooosh." Let it all out. Do this a few times with your normal breathing pattern, then slow it down. Count to three as you inhale, hold for three, and then again count to three as you exhale. Focus on the air coming into and going out of your body. Visualize the air as a white light, a beam of energy that comes into your lungs, into your belly, and branches off into veins with its brightness cleansing everything in its path. When you exhale, the dim, grayer "exhaust" is dispelled in the opposite motion, but exiting through the mouth.

As you feel yourself calm and relax, go ahead and slow your breathing down even more by increasing your count to four. Give yourself several inhalations and exhalations at the four count, then slow your breathing down a touch more by increasing the count to five. Continue to breathe at this pace for several minutes. Allow yourself a full song of this deep relaxation breathing along with the visualization of the cleansing white light. If you are comfortable slowing the breathing down again, do so. Reach the place where you feel relaxed, almost hypnotized by your own breathing, but not struggling for air.

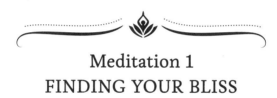

Meditation 1
FINDING YOUR BLISS

Session 1

Set your mood. (This includes your lighting, candles, incense, decorations, protective circle, etc.)

Write your intention down in your journal. For this meditation, you will be looking into what has given you the greatest joy in your life so far.

Complete your pre-meditation breathing exercise.

Think back to the earliest in your childhood you remember. What are some memories you have of pure happiness? What caused you to feel that way? Is there a special place you find happiness? Certain people who have brought you joy time and time again? Fast forward through your life to another happy moment. This may be a few months later or a few years later; don't concern yourself as much with precise timelines as you do with finding those most perfect moments to work with. Answer the same question: what was the root of your happiness? Try to remember how you felt at the time. When you are happy now, do you still feel the same way? If not, what is different? Fast forward in time again to another happy moment. Explore your feelings at each of your stops. Is there an overall theme to things that make up your happiest moments, or are they more random? How have those moments shaped who you are now? Spend as much time in this meditation as you want, simply revisiting those moments in your life that gave you the greatest joy and answering the same questions about them.

When you are ready to finish, spend one last moment feeling as much of that bliss as you can, all at once. Hold on to it for a moment and then let it go with peace.

Spend some time journaling about the events you experienced and what you were able to feel.

If working with a partner, during the meditation they may guide you by asking you to find an event and then asking you the questions about it. You will want to be doing this with your cannabis sessions, so if you want to do it the same way "sober," that is up to you, but again, not necessary.

This meditation is about exploring what has made you the happiest throughout your life, not only to remind you of what made you happy, but to relive the feelings and emotions that you felt at those moments—to see how fully you can experience those same emotions now, many years later. One of the important goals in these first few meditations is to be able to show you the difference in how you *feel* between aided and unaided meditations. Therefore, this first meditation is helping us set a baseline for your experiences. Cannabis-aided meditations allow you to *feel* on a completely different level than what you are used to. Everything is far more intense. Using happy times in your life to show you the difference is fun but—at the same time—highly enlightening. The amount of cannabis you use is also going to affect how intense those feelings can become. A light high will not be the same as a peak experience. This is a fun meditation to practice several times using different doses to see how they compare to one another.

Sessions 2 and 3

You will conduct these two sessions in the exact same manner as you did session one. Each time you perform the meditation, go back to the same moments you chose before. Look for any details you may have missed the first time.

After you finish the meditation the second time, again write about it in your journal. Only after you have written about it should you go back and read the notes from your first session. Then you can add anything else you want to include.

At the end of session three, do the same thing: write about your meditation, then go back and reread your notes from sessions one and two. Again, document any changes or new information you may come across in your working.

Additional Journal Questions:
1. As you perform the meditation more times, do your feelings about the event change at all?
2. If so, how?
3. Does your emotional response seem to be stronger, or has it lessened somehow?
4. If it has changed, how?

Session 4

This session will be the first time you combine cannabis with your visualization, so be sure to include your dosage information. You don't need to get completely stoned off your rocker; in fact, I would rather you didn't! Let's start slow, with just enough cannabis to have you feeling good. You should be relaxed, but not too sedated. With the next two sessions, you will be increasing your dosage. You also need to consider how much time you plan on practicing. If you took ten minutes to do the meditation sober, allow yourself the same amount of time (and perhaps a little longer) to complete it aided. If you went longer and know that you will need to keep consuming cannabis to maintain your state, then have that prepared and ready to go.

We will be following the same format as before, while adding in dosing. The steps will be:

1. Set your mood (turn on music, light candles or incense, set decorations, etc.)
2. Journal documentation: time, dosage information, intention
3. Consume cannabis
4. Get into position and begin pre-meditation breathing exercise

This meditation has a very simple premise to it, so you may not need much guiding from your partner, but you do have to keep communicating so they know you aren't just drifting off. With these shorter, easier meditations, the unaided practice meditations also help you to learn the meditation. Depending on how high you are, though, you may forget what you were doing. This is when a partner needs to speak up and steer you back to the task at hand. For new users of cannabis, getting off track is easy!

It may take some trial and error figuring out how best to work with each other, and that's no problem either. Working at it together, you will find a balance that works for you. The focus of this session is twofold.

One, this is your first real chance to be focused on a specific topic while under the influence of cannabis. Take your time, relax, and enjoy it. Remember to talk to your partner about what you are feeling. Two, you go back to those same events as before. Can you visualize them more intently? Do you feel the same? Do you feel different? Allow your partner to assist you by reminding you to talk about your feelings.

How you feel this first time is going to be extremely dependent on your dosing and how it affects you. You may not feel much at all; if you don't, go ahead and increase your dosage and be sure to document it. Give yourself some more time—up to twenty minutes—to see if your experience intensifies or not. If it doesn't, go ahead and dose again.

Quick Tip: While you want to focus on these past events that brought you joy, if you try to focus too hard while on cannabis, you may end up hyper-focused, which can diminish your high and cause you to focus more on the events than on the feelings associated with those events. It takes a bit of practice to learn how to walk the path and be able to do what you want to do. Our meditations call for relaxation and focus, but both with moderation.

If you can complete both tasks your first time around, congratulations! If not, don't worry about it. You can repeat the meditation as many times as you need to. I recommend the three times so that each time you can increase your dosing to bring you closer and closer to a peak experience. If you do not hit a peak experience, don't worry! Again, this is practice, and practice doesn't have to be perfect. Every time you do not hit a peak experience, you learn more about what it takes to get there. You will know what is out of balance because you can *feel* it. This is one reason why the communication with your partner is important, so they can help you find exactly what you need to hit a peak experience. The first time I hit a peak I thought it was totally amazing, but I also had no clue what it had taken me to get there, making it difficult to duplicate the process. You must pay attention to how the cannabis is affecting you and learn how to ride it to get you to your destination. Don't fight it, but instead give in and let it wash over you.

When you have completed the meditation, be sure to write about your experience and read over your partner's notes. Use this information to plan for session five.

Session 5

Using the information you have gained up to this point, set yourself up to complete session five the same as you did session four. Your only difference should be the amount of cannabis you consume. (If you do find you need to make changes in seating, lighting, or music, always feel free to do that. I'm only referring to differences in our procedure here.)

Increase your dosage (being sure to document it) and repeat the meditation from there. How does this new dosage affect how the meditation works for you? Has your view of these events changed? Are you able to experience the joy in a more "firsthand" experience? Does the meditation seem more "real"? Are you able to tap into other aspects of the environment where the event took place?

Here are some examples. Perhaps your experience is at a beach. Can you hear the waves? Smell the water in the air? Feel the heat of the sun? The grit of the sand? Can you smell the hotdogs cooking nearby on a grill? Can you taste the blue raspberry slushie you slurped down with a straw? Can you feel the ice beads as they travel down your esophagus? Use all your senses to bring this experience as much to life as you can. Try to put yourself back into that exact moment in time. We often rely on our sight, but the sense of smell is very potent in bringing back memories. Combining all your senses to recreate the moment will help intensify the effect. The cannabis also helps to intensify the effects by boosting the signals from your other senses, which in turn allows the cannabis to work even better. That's the thing with cannabis; if you allow it to work, it will.

Throughout this session, again, be sure to communicate with your partner. Tell them everything you possibly can about this meditation. At the end, write about it in your journal, read your partner's notes, and then add any additional comments you want to make.

Additional Journal Questions:
1. As you perform the meditation more often, do your feelings about the event change at all?
2. If so, how?
3. Does your emotional response seem to be stronger, or has it lessened somehow?
4. If it has changed, how?

Session 6

By now you should not only have a firm grasp on this meditation, but you should be getting a good idea of how to work along with the cannabis to create the mindset and then follow through for your meditations to be successful. If you think you need more practice, feel free to continue performing this meditation even after this session. The next meditation, "finding your space," will be similar in scope, but may also require a bit of imagination depending on your real-life experiences.

In this session, you will again start off with an increased dose. How did session five go for you? If you feel you are ready for a larger dose than you used in session five, go for it. Continue to dose to maintain or elevate your high as needed. Continue to communicate with your partner regarding your feelings, emotions, and what you can take in from your other senses. Go back to those points in life you have been revisiting. When you are ready, increase your dose again. Will yourself to *be* in those moments of your bliss. Allow yourself to go there. Let yourself get lost in the moment. If you do not feel a very strong awareness of "now" and everything around you, you have not yet hit a peak. That is okay; you will get there!

Continue to increase your dose as much as you feel comfortable doing. Remember to use your partner to help maintain your comfort. Do you need water? I often find myself feeling dehydrated during and after a peak experience (mainly cotton mouth). Do you want the lights out? I highly prefer very dim to no light for a peak experience.

When you hit a peak, you feel unlimited and uninhibited. The world around you stands still and time itself seems a foreign concept. A peak experience may feel hours long, but instead only lasts ten minutes. Eventually, you will learn how (by trial and error, and possibly by intuition) to extend your peak experience with proper dosing. It reminds me of when TV shows or movies show witches freezing time. While time is stopped the witch can move around and see things from angles that wouldn't otherwise be feasible, giving the witch new and interesting viewpoints. Hitting a peak experience is very similar. It allows you to see time differently and look at situations from a different point of view. This is the gift of cannabis; it is what allows us to use it to heal ourselves mentally and emotionally, making us more whole and complete.

Once you can hit a peak while performing this meditation, you will discover just how much more intensely you can experience the emotions you felt before. It's like a sliding scale from one to ten. While a casual memory may rate around a two, that same memory focused on during a meditation may rate around a five in intensity. Once you add cannabis into the mix, you start feeling an intensity level of eight. When you hit a peak experience, your intensity level registers at an eleven+ because you had no idea that kind of emotional outpouring was even possible.

Finish this meditation in a way that makes you comfortable. If you haven't hit a peak with it yet, you can continue to work with it, or move on to meditation two. Meditation two is going to focus on creating your own personal safe space. This may be a place you create from scratch or one you already know of but want to spruce up a bit with your own imagination. You may find it beneficial to move on to meditation two for a little imagination usage and then come back to try meditation one again. Remember to journal any thoughts from this meditation and review notes from your partner to finish out your session.

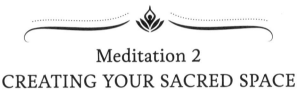

Meditation 2
CREATING YOUR SACRED SPACE

Session 1

Set your mood.

Write your intention down in your journal. For this meditation you are creating your own sacred space, a space to feel completely at peace and at one with the universe.

Complete your pre-meditation breathing exercise.

Imagine what your perfect sanctuary would look like. You may include an entire setting, such as your ideal room in your ideal home in your ideal location, or you may make it more concise and focus on a smaller area instead. It may be a forest glade or a spot on the beach. If the place makes you feel safe, at peace, and in harmony with the universe, then you are building the right location. What does it look like? Where is it? Is it a real place you have been to or would like to visit in the future? Is it a make-believe location from a book, a movie, or your own imagination? Is it in this time period? Perhaps your ideal safe place is the Isle of Avalon, or even Atlantis. See it in your mind with as much detail as you can. Spend as much time in this meditation as you want, discovering and exploring your safe space. If you are working with a partner, be sure to communicate to them what the space is like. Be sure to describe it in your journal to finish your session.

My sacred space is nothing like what I had originally intended. It has evolved over time, and yours may do the same as well. Allow it to change as needed. The physical aspects of the location are not as important as the feelings it evokes. I begin in my own sacred space and often end in what reminds me of a bubble. I am floating in a space resembling a picture of a galaxy. Different colored energy swirls around me in different patterns. It's a place where I can reach out and touch the stars. I am a physical presence, and at the same time, I am not. I am both at the same time. Yours may end up being similar, or it may be something else entirely. Your knowledge base, beliefs, and overall mindset will make a huge impact on your sacred space.

Sessions 2 and 3

In these two sessions you will again go back to your safe space and explore it as much as you can. What about this place gives you peace? How does it make you feel connected to the universe? What do you hear? Smell? Taste? When you come here, can you feel the same joy or bliss you conjured in meditation one? Try to find that bliss, and feel it here in your sacred, safe place. Combine the two parts into one, pulling the joy into your space so you can tap into it anytime you are here. Immerse yourself as deeply into this world as you can. Spend as much time in these meditations as you need. Describe it to your partner and in your journal with as much detail as you can to finish these sessions.

Session 4

As a reminder, here is the format we are following:

1. Set mood

2. Journal documentations: time, dosage information, intention

3. Consume cannabis

4. Get into position and begin pre-meditation breathing exercise

Your dose should be similar to what you used for the previous meditation's session five. If you felt the dosage had been off, either too little or too much, you can adjust it now. Your goal again is to start slow and increase the dosage each time to fully emphasize the differences, and so you can more easily track your progress. Once you get more accustomd to practicing like this, you can increase the dosages even more at the onset of each session.

Take yourself back to the sacred safe place you created. How does it appear different to you now with the aid of cannabis? Is it more vibrant? Can you immerse yourself into your self-constructed environment more easily and more deeply? Can you feel yourself there? What do you see? Smell? Hear? Reach out with your senses to pull yourself in more deeply. Can you connect with your bliss more easily? If you hit a peak experience, what do you find different about your space? Throughout your session, continue to communicate with your partner. Close your session by journaling about the experience.

Sessions 5 and 6

If you have already hit a peak experience, use these two sessions to repeat the meditation in the same way as session four, and try to hit a peak experience once again. Once you get the hang of hitting a peak, it will be far easier to hit them much more often, but you must get there first.

If you have not been able to hit a peak experience yet, we are going to work on increasing your dosage to see if you can do so during sessions five and six. You may also need to work more on connecting to your bliss while stoned. Open your awareness and let your partner know if there is a way they can help remove a blockage. Do you know what is holding you back? Are you nervous? Allowing the cannabis to work and relax you will also allow the cannabis to help you see what it is you are missing while making these connections.

Begin session five with a higher dose than session four. Give yourself several minutes to begin relaxing into the high, then dose again. Allow yourself to relax more. Let yourself sink into the high. Continue working on your breathing as you are dosing; it will help the cannabis work. Dose again if necessary. You may need several doses to allow yourself to fully relax into a high. You may need several doses more to achieve a peak experience.

Transition to your sacred space and raise your awareness to your surroundings. Continue using your senses to explore the environment all around you. Explore the connection you feel to the environment. Be sure to talk to your partner about what you feel and experience. Your partner should ask questions when needed to ensure that you stay on your journey and don't mentally wander off and forget the meditation. It can be difficult to stay on task; your partner is invaluable in helping you learn how to redirect yourself to the meditation at hand instead of veering off onto tangents. There will be a time for that later, but first you want to learn how to control where your mind focuses.

Work on increasing dosage, maintaining a high, and opening your awareness to the sacred space you have created. Allowing these things to happen makes it easier to let go of your inhibitions. Once you let go, achieving a peak is possible.

Continue to work on these aspects as you progress through sessions five and six. You may repeat this meditation as many times as you want if you still feel a need. Otherwise, it's time to move on to meeting the divine.

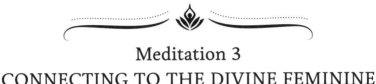

Meditation 3
CONNECTING TO THE DIVINE FEMININE

It is the flower buds of the female cannabis plants that are so rich in THC and other cannabinoids (other parts of the plant do contain cannabinoids, but not high concentrations of THC). Because of this natural connection to the Divine Feminine, I do feel it is easier (for me at least) to connect to the Feminine than to the Masculine, but being female myself may also make it that way.

You may want to envision this meditation as somewhat similar to drawing down the moon. The goddess you work with does not have to enter your body to speak through you, but that can be done in later workings. For now, you only want to call the goddess into your sacred space to be able to commune with her.

This can be very difficult for people without the aid of cannabis or other entheogens, so do not be discouraged if the three sessions without aid simply don't allow you to make the connection you wish to make. Other people have a great experience with this and will have no issues with it at all. Each of us has different talents.

If doing this on your own, you may use the script if you would like, by recording yourself reading it. If you are working with a partner, your partner will be able to use the script to walk you through. Whoever does the reading should be sure to do it slowly, allowing plenty of time between each sentence. Use your best judgment, keeping at least a minute between each sentence.

A word on "speaking" with deities and/or guides: When in a meditation I say something like "tell your deity guide what you need," or even recommend greetings and farewells. Your communication does not have to be verbal if you don't want it to be. When you join with deity in a peak experience, you understand the meaning of telepathy or "mind meld." Your deity, your guide, knows your thoughts as you have them, and you are completely aware and comfortable that they know them. However, if you do speak out loud it does give your partner more information.

Session 1

Set your mood. If you have pictures, statutes, or other goddess representations, you will want to add these to your physical space to help set your mood. Be sure to include several different ones.

Write your intention in your journal. For this meditation you will be asking the Divine Feminine to meet with you in your created sacred space. While it may be tempting to request the presence of a specific deity, for now I ask that you be open and accepting to whatever aspect of divinity presents itself. While you may normally work with a specific pantheon, please use this time of exploration to see who presents herself to you.

Complete your pre-meditation breathing exercise.

Script

Journey back to your sacred space.
Let the feeling of peace and awareness wash over you.
Reach out with your heart and mind to find the bliss
and contentment held here in this space for you.

Give yourself a few minutes to get to your space. If you are working with a partner, you can tell your partner when you are there and ready to move on—this is part of why working with a partner is so much easier than working on your own! These first several lines we will use to open each meditation. This helps set the ritual journey you take on each time you start your quest for a peak experience.

Open your awareness to everything around you.
What do you see?
What do you feel?
In your own mind, ask the Divine Feminine to
approach you, to enter your sacred space.
Invite her to join with you.
Open yourself to any and all possibilities.

Again, if this doesn't work for you now, do not be discouraged. Allow yourself to be open and welcoming to any deity who shows up, but if no one does, that is okay; after all, it's only your first try! If you do not make a connection after about twenty minutes of trying, end your meditation, but be sure to still write about what did happen. If an aspect of the Divine Feminine does enter your sacred space, continue with the meditation as follows, again leaving plenty of time between each question.

Who has come to meet with you? If you do
not recognize her, ask for her name.
Describe how she looks.
What does it feel like to be in her presence?
Does she have a message for you? If so, what is it?
When you are ready, graciously thank the deity
for appearing to you and say goodbye.

Finish up your session by writing about your experience and reading over any notes from your partner, if you had one. Answer the questions from your meditation in your journal.

Sessions 2 and 3

These two sessions will be conducted exactly the same as session one. If you were not able to make a connection, try changing your setting up a little. Adjust the lighting, try different music or different incense. While these things may not seem as important, they do play a major role in your state of mind. Give yourself more time during the meditation if you feel you need it. Before each of these sessions, be sure to document any changes you made. After the sessions, document if the changes helped, along with any other new information you obtained while working through them.

If you were able to make a connection the first time, perform these two sessions in the same manner, allowing whomever wants to come through to do so. You may find a different deity comes through each time, or perhaps it is the same one each time. If this does happen, the message this deity has for you is obviously quite important. Be sure to listen with an open heart and mind to receive the message clearly.

Another quick reminder: A large part of the focus of these meditations is to be able to see the difference between being aided and unaided by cannabis. Even if you can't make the connection now, you still have a good chance of doing so when you do use cannabis to help you get there. Each time you perform the meditation, you are also learning it and making it easier to perform, giving you a good foundation to work with when you do add cannabis into the mix. There is no such thing as "failure" when doing these meditations, as everything adds up to prep work for when you do have a "success."

Session 4

As a reminder, here is the format we are following:

1. Set mood
2. Journal documentation: time, dosage information, intention
3. Consume cannabis
4. Get into position and begin pre-meditation breathing exercise

By now you've had a bit of experience with dosing and have a better idea of what works for you. If you aren't having any issues—awesome! Keep doing things the way you have been. If you haven't hit a peak experience yet, you need to increase your dosing again and perhaps make changes to your setup. One of the most common reasons for not hitting a peak experience is your mindset. Some people fight the feeling because it is so new. You may experience some negative reactions before hitting a peak (nausea, dry mouth, possibly anxiety). You need to push through and persevere. Remind yourself that whatever feelings you have are normal and they will pass. Allow any doubt, fear, or anxiety to dissolve. Keep working toward feeling awareness of everything around you and letting that be your guide. I can't stress enough that you must *allow* it to happen. For people who like to be in and keep control, it can be difficult to let go. Even after you think you have let go, you will realize you are still holding yourself back. In fact, this may happen to you several times. The first time I hit a peak experience, it wasn't planned; in fact, the first several times I did *try* to hit one, I realized I was trying too hard and not letting all my walls down. Even when I thought they were down, as I inhaled more THC, I could still feel barriers around me. My mind wandered to "what if" questions. My mind likes to race a lot. It takes a significant amount of effort on my part to stop that and to allow the THC to do its job and lower all barriers and blockages in my way.

Allow your partner to guide you through the script, dosing as you feel you need it. Your partner should give you plenty of time—several minutes if needed—between each statement or question.

Script

Journey back to your sacred space.
Let the feeling of peace and awareness wash over you.
Reach out with your heart and mind to find the bliss
and contentment held here in this space for you.
Open your awareness to everything around you.
What do you see?
What do you feel?
In your own mind, ask the Divine Feminine to
approach you, to enter your sacred space.
Invite her to join with you.
Open yourself to any and all possibilities.
Who has come to meet with you? If you do not
recognize her, ask for her name.
Describe how she looks.
What does it feel like to be in her presence?
Does she have a message for you? If so, what is it?
When you are ready, graciously thank the deity
for appearing to you and say goodbye.

Finish up your session by writing about your experience and reading over any notes from your partner. If you feel you need to hear more from your partner, let them know that. They can repeat your instructions several times if that works better for you. For many people, the less outside talking there is the easier it is for them to shut off the physical presence and focus on the spiritual presence instead. Still, others need more guidance. This is a matter of your own personal preference, so if you are still having issues, try changing up just how much your partner guides you.

By the time you make it through this meditation, you should have enough practice under your belt to be able to judge your situation and know what you need in terms of comfort and dosing. In sessions five and six, we are going to extend the script to give you more interaction with the deity who comes to visit.

Finish your session by journaling and reviewing the notes from your partner.

Sessions 5 and 6

You should have the schedule ingrained now, so I won't continue to repeat it. If you need to, you can refer back to earlier meditations in this chapter for that information.

Once you are all dosed and ready to go, your partner can begin guiding you through the extended script.

Script

Journey back to your sacred space.
Let the feelings of peace and awareness wash over you.
Allow all tension to fall away.
Reach out with your heart and mind to find the bliss
and contentment held here in this space for you.
Open your awareness to everything around you.
What do you see?
What do you feel?
What do you hear?
In your own mind, ask the Divine Feminine to
approach you, to enter your sacred space.
Invite her to join with you.
Open yourself to any and all possibilities.

Who has come to meet with you? If you do
not recognize her, ask for her name.
Describe how she looks.
What does it feel like to be in her presence?
Does she have a message for you? If so, what is it?
In your mind, reach your hand out to her.
Feel her energy surging around you and through you.
Describe the sensation as best you can.
When you are ready, graciously thank the deity
for appearing to you, and say goodbye.

In your journal writing, be sure to discuss the differences you are finding between aided and unaided meditations. Are you able to feel the difference in intensity? Are you finding yourself able to go deeper into your meditations? Are you having difficulties? If so, what are they?

As you get more proficient at this meditation, you may use it in different ways, including drawing down the specific goddess you want to work with or would like help from. Learning to connect with the goddess in this way is truly fulfilling. You can also use it to call on any guides you want to work with.

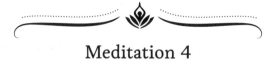

Meditation 4
CONNECTING TO THE DIVINE MASCULINE

While it may be easier to connect with the Divine Feminine due to the nature of the cannabis plant, that does not mean it is impossible to connect with the Divine Masculine. The first time I connected with a male deity I was surprised, as he was not who I was seeking for assistance. I had been working with Cerridwen, Blodeuwedd, and the Morrigan on different issues when one night Pan appeared unexpectedly with a message for me. I was amazed at how much I could feel the difference between him and the female deities I had previously worked with in a peak experience. While these three goddesses all have very distinct energies, the energy from Pan was, well, far more masculine. There was no doubt I had made a strong connection with an entity I had not encountered in a peak experience previously. This is one of the joys of a peak experience; the intensity of the connection makes it unique each and every time. This meditation will be very similar, script-wise (and process-wise), as the meditation for connecting to the Divine Feminine.

Be sure to set up your area with some pictures or statues of different aspects of the Divine Masculine.

Session 1

Set your mood.

Write your intention down in your journal. For this meditation you will be asking the Divine Masculine to meet with you in your created sacred space. Again, do not ask for a specific deity; wait and see who comes to you.

Complete your pre-meditation breathing exercise.

Script

Journey back to your sacred space.
Let the feeling of peace and awareness wash over you.
Reach out with your heart and mind to find the
bliss and contentment held here in this space for you.

Give yourself a few minutes to get to your space. If you are working with a partner, you can tell your partner when you are there and ready to move on.

> *Open your awareness to everything around you.*
> *What do you see?*
> *What do you feel?*
> *In your own mind, ask the Divine Masculine*
> *to approach you, to enter your sacred space.*
> *Invite him to join with you.*
> *Open yourself to any and all possibilities.*
> *Who has come to meet with you? If you*
> *do not recognize him, ask for his name.*
> *Describe how he looks.*
> *What does it feel like to be in his presence?*
> *Does he have a message for you? If so, what is it?*
> *When you are ready, graciously thank the deity*
> *for appearing to you and say goodbye.*

Finish up your session by writing about your experience and reading over any notes from your partner if you used one.

Sessions 2 and 3

If you were not able to make a connection, try changing your setting up a little. Adjust the lighting, try different music or different incense. Perhaps you might want to try something with a more masculine vibe to it. Before each of these sessions, document any changes you made. After the sessions, document if the changes helped, along with any other new information you obtained while working through them.

If you were able to make a connection, perform these two meditations in the same manner as the first one, allowing whoever wants to come through to do so.

Session 4

Allow your partner to guide you through the script, dosing as you feel you need it. Your partner should give you plenty of time—several minutes—between each statement or question.

Finish up your session by writing about your experience and reading over any notes from your partner. Be sure to read back over the meditation so you can answer the questions in your journal.

Sessions 5 and 6

Once you are all dosed and ready to go, your partner can begin guiding you through the extended script.

Script

Journey back to your sacred space.
Let the feeling of peace and awareness wash over you.
Allow all tension to fall away.
Reach out with your heart and mind to find the bliss
and contentment held here in this space for you.
Open your awareness to everything around you.
What do you see?
What do you feel?
What do you hear?
In your own mind, ask the Divine Masculine to approach
you, to enter your sacred space.
Invite him to join with you.
Open yourself to any and all possibilities.

Who has come to meet with you?
If you do not recognize him, ask for his name.
Describe how he looks.
What does it feel like to be in his presence?
Does he have a message for you? If so, what is it?
In your mind, reach your hand out to him.
Feel his energy surging around you and through you.
Describe the sensation as best you can.
When you are ready, graciously thank the deity for appearing
to you, and say goodbye.

As you get more proficient at this meditation, you may use it in different ways, including drawing down the specific god you want to work with or would like help from. You can also use it to call on any guides you want to work with.

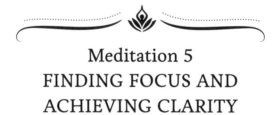

Meditation 5
FINDING FOCUS AND
ACHIEVING CLARITY

One of the biggest misconceptions about using cannabis is that it makes you fuzzy or unable to focus. This isn't always true. The nature of cannabis can make you forgetful, if you are not channeling and focusing the energy. This is one of the reasons you are using a partner. But, used with the correct mindset, cannabis can actually allow you to become hyper-focused. You must be sure to channel and direct the focus where you want it. Think of cannabis as a doorway that will lead wherever you want it to go. If you want to veg out and be a couch potato, cannabis has your back. But if you want to use the very same cannabis to focus and look deeply into the presence of your soul in the universe … well, cannabis has your back for that too. This is also going to be affected by the strain you use. For clarity work, a sativa or sativa-dominant hybrid may be best for you.

Have you ever wished you could relive a moment of your life but do everything differently? While it may not be full-blown devastating remorse you feel (or it could be!), maybe there is something that has nagged at you for a while, or you were never quite sure what happened. What went wrong for things to turn out the way they did. Perhaps it is a moment you have had a difficult time getting past.

This meditation is created to journey back to those types of moments and see them through a different eye, the eye of someone who can look more objectively and thoroughly at all sides of the situation. It is going to give you clarity over the situation, so you may acknowledge it, heal from it, and move on from it.

You may find this meditation difficult to do unaided. That is perfectly natural. Even when it doesn't seem like you have had a successful meditation session, it's important to remember that there is always something to be learned from it. In the cases of these meditations, if you do not feel like you are getting very far on your own in the unaided sessions, there is nothing wrong with that all. At the very least you are learning the meditation, so it is easier for you to follow along with when you are under the influence.

Sessions 1–3

Set your mood.

Write your intention down in your journal. For this meditation, either choose a specific moment you want to go back to or ask your guide to take you to the moment they choose, for you to see it through their eyes so you can get clarity over the situation. This meditation can be repeated over and over for any situation you need clarity about.

Complete your pre-meditation breathing exercise.

Script

Journey back to your sacred space.
Let the feeling of peace and awareness wash over you.
Allow all tension to fall away.
Reach out with your heart and mind to find the bliss
and contentment held here in this space for you.
Open your awareness to everything around you.
Spend a moment immersed in the pleasure of the
connection you feel with the universe.
Feel the energy around you.
Allow it to flow through you.
When you are ready, call upon the deity or
guide you wish to work with.
When they arrive, feel their energy stream
around you and breeze through you.
Enjoy their presence.
Send your energy out to combine with
theirs in your sacred space.
Revel in the pleasure of their presence.
When you are ready, tell your guest
(specific name if desired) what your need is.
Allow the request to be felt through you and your guide.
When ready, open your mind's eye to the time
and place where you need to be.
You are inside of yourself, but outside too.
You are in the air. In the environment all around you.
You are in everything and everyone around you.

Your guide is here with you, showing you the way.
Replay the chosen scene around you.
Not in front of you, but around you.
See yourself in the center looking out, then outside looking in.
See it from the eyes of the others involved.
See it from the viewpoint of your guide—all seeing, all knowing.
What does your guide want you to see?
What have you been missing, or
hiding from yourself or others?
What have you been neglecting to see?
Spend as much time as you need here.
When you are ready, thank and dismiss your guide.

Finish your session by journaling about the experience. Describe the situation and what you can now see differently. It may take several times per incident to learn the "lesson" to give yourself complete clarity over the situation.

Sessions 4–6

These sessions will be conducted in the same way as sessions one through three, but with the addition of the cannabis.

By now you are probably getting a good idea of how much more intense and realistic these meditations feel when they are aided. You will also find that they are far easier to perform.

This meditation is an important stepping stone to some of the other meditations we will do later on. Not only does it teach you how to find clarity in a specific situation, but it teaches you how to focus and direct your energy into specific memories and events. These are skills that will come in handy in your workings to come. As always, at the end of each session, add your thoughts to your journal.

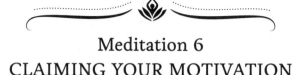

Meditation 6
CLAIMING YOUR MOTIVATION

Motivation can be a tricky subject to work with. Sometimes we get lazy. Sometimes we like to procrastinate. Some of us do it far better and far more often than others. We are always told to "get motivated" or we say we "need to find some motivation" in order to get things done. But what does this really mean?

What it means is that we must find what drives us, what inspires us, what excites us, what propels us to move forward. In other words, we really need to ask ourselves "What is in it for me?" This is really what it comes down to. Even in doing for others, we are fulfilling a need within ourselves while fulfilling a need for someone else. This isn't as selfish as it sounds. We do need to meet our own needs in order to meet the needs of others. So, finding your motivation is really about finding what inspires you. It's about asking "What do I get out of it?" It's about finding what you need to feel in order to want to do something. Money can be a great motivator because of the buying power and safety net it can give. The key here is the power and safety net— not the money. I do a lot of volunteering with the homeless. One of my motivating factors is my own security. I was homeless briefly many years in the past, and the uncertainty of it was crushing. I do not ever want to feel that way again, nor do I like others having to feel it. Helping others has helped me to heal from that time in my life.

This meditation is going to help you find what needs and what insecurities you have that can be turned to motivate you in other areas of your life. This can help you be more productive while healing past wounds.

Sessions 1–3

Set your mood.

Write your intention down in your journal. For this meditation you will look for what emotional needs you have that can be used to motivate you in other areas of your life.

Complete your pre-meditation breathing exercise.

Script

Journey back to your sacred space.
Let the feeling of peace and awareness wash over you.
Allow all tension to fall away.
Reach out with your heart and mind to find the
bliss and contentment held here in this space for you.
Open your awareness to everything around you.
Spend a moment immersed in the pleasure of
the connection you feel with the universe.
Feel the energy around you.
Allow it to flow through you.
When you are ready, call upon the deity
or guide you wish to work with.
When they arrive, feel their energy stream
around you and breeze through you.
Enjoy their presence.
Send your energy out to combine
with theirs in your sacred space.
Revel in the pleasure of their presence.
When you are ready, ask your guide to
show you your greatest need.
Allow the request to be felt through you and your guide.
What do you need in order to feel whole?
What makes you feel loved and complete?

Do you feel this is missing from your life?
Allow yourself to feel whatever it is you need.
Let your emotions flow through you and around you.
You don't need to do anything about these feelings.
You don't need to fix them. Just allow yourself to feel them.
Acknowledge that they are there and are a part of you.
Spend as much time as you need here.
When you are ready, thank and dismiss your guide.

Finish your session by journaling about the experience.

Sessions 4–6

Conduct these sessions just as you did the first three, but with the addition of cannabis. Knowing what you need in order to feel more complete is another step toward making yourself whole and raising your spiritual vibration. When you journal about this meditation, brainstorm about ways you can meet the needs you have. We often count on other people to attempt to make ourselves feel whole. Truth is, no one else can do it for us. This is something we must do for ourselves.

Checking In

By the time you complete this meditation, you should have a good foundation to be able to see and compare the differences between unaided and aided sessions. If you are finding that the three unaided sessions aren't giving you unique results, go ahead and cut them down to one or two times before adding the cannabis. Every now and then we have to stop and reexamine our practice to see if there are changes we should be making. What has been beneficial to you so far? What has seemed like a waste of time? What can you do to make your practice more practical?

The rest of the solitary meditations I will not be breaking down by sessions. You will now decide how many sessions you want/need of each; just remember to do them at least once before moving on to the next, with no skipping around.

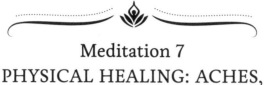

Meditation 7
PHYSICAL HEALING: ACHES, PAINS, BREAKS, AND SPRAINS

Meditation, visualization, Reiki, and other forms of energy work can be extremely beneficial when used for healing, both physically and emotionally. We all need healing at some point in our lives. Whether it's for a small inconvenience or a life-altering illness, learning to use our own energy—along with energy from the universe and our deities—to assist in healing is essential. Doctors will often tell you that attitude is a large part of healing, I believe this to be true. The act of meditating through your illness is a step in the direction of better health.

This is a longer meditation and you will need plenty of time between each statement. Plan on spending at least a half an hour in this meditation. Drawing it out to forty-five minutes is ideal.

Set your mood.

Write your intention down in your journal. For this meditation you will be focusing on healing a physical ailment, so be sure to include what it is you will be working on. This can be anything from a cold to a sprained ankle, a headache, or something more serious, like a chronic illness. If you have no ailments, this can be used simply to promote good health and will still work as a cleansing.

Complete your pre-meditation breathing exercise.

Script

Journey back to your sacred space.
Let the feeling of peace and awareness wash over you.
Allow all tension to fall away.
Reach out with your heart and mind to find the
bliss and contentment held here in this space for you.
Open your awareness to everything around you.
Spend a moment immersed in the pleasure
of the connection you feel with the universe.
Feel the energy around you.
Allow it to flow through you.
When you are ready, call upon the
deity you wish to work with.
When they arrive, feel their energy stream
around you and breeze through you.
Enjoy their presence.
Send your energy out to combine with
theirs in your sacred space.
Revel in the pleasure of their presence.
When you are ready, tell your deity or guide (you may
insert a specific name here) what aid and comfort you seek.
As you inhale, imagine you are breathing in the
energy radiated by both yourself and your deity.
See this energy as a swirling white light,
flowing into your body, through your lungs,
and into your veins, traveling throughout your body.
Allow the energy to flow all across
your body, cleansing as it goes.
Take your time.
Direct and focus the energy light to
the areas that need healing.

Allow it to spiral, scrubbing away the
negativity of your affliction.
See and feel yourself being cleansed and healed by the light.
Spend as much time here as you desire.
When you are ready, thank your deity for
their presence, for their love, for their aid.
Bid them farewell.

Finish your session by journaling about the experience.

As someone who has endured pain the vast majority of her life, I love to attest to the healing abilities of cannabis. While CBD has become the new rage for pain relief, it really does work best when combined with THC. It works even better when you can use the THC to help promote your own self-healing through introspection and visualization in the depths of a peak experience meditation.

Because this meditation is longer, you will need to be sure to keep dosing to maintain your high or peak. Your partner will also need to give you plenty of time in between each statement. When you add cannabis to your meditations, especially longer meditations, they can be stretched out quite easily. Your brain is entertained and able to hyper-focus on the meditation. Without cannabis, you may find your mind wandering off the task at hand, but with cannabis you are brought more into the moment of NOW, where other distractions cease to exist. If you spent thirty to forty-five minutes in this meditation without cannabis, expect to spend forty-five to sixty minutes with it. Finish your session by journaling about the experience.

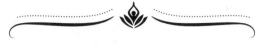

Meditation 8
EMOTIONAL HEALING:
MAKING PEACE WITH THE PAST

While you may know some precise areas where you need emotional healing, other aspects may be hidden from you. These meditations, particularly when you are working with cannabis, will help unveil masked issues you need to deal with. You may not be able to uncover too much without the assistance of cannabis, but don't worry—the plant is capable of bringing down walls you didn't even know you had.

I'm not going to lie, this can get painful. It's the equivalent of holding up a mirror and suddenly seeing your faults for the first time. Not physical faults, but deep-down hidden faults. On the positive side, you will be seeing yourself in a new light, as if through the eyes of another person. This not only gives you new information about yourself, but it gives you the opportunity to make changes in your life. For empaths, this meditation may feel even more potent, as you will be seeing for yourself how someone else sees your emotional damage, and quite possibly feeling the viewer's emotions along with your own. What I mean is this: if you wronged someone and didn't realize it, not only will you have a reckoning about the committed wrongdoing, but you will be able to feel how that person felt in response to it. Cannabis will intensify the emotion of this meditation. Be ready for this. If after three sessions without cannabis you don't feel ready to use cannabis with this meditation, don't. Perform it a few more times, but don't go on to the next meditation until you have completed this one.

Remember, our minds and our guides and deities all have something in common: they protect us. Sometimes our minds hide things from us that would hurt us, in order to protect us. You may learn things or remember things you don't like, but this is all part of the healing process. You are safe. The guide or deity you choose to work with will be with you. You are not alone. Our protectors also know not to give us more than we can handle at any one time. You won't get dumped on with every bad thing you've ever done at once. What needs to be revealed to you will be revealed to you, and at exactly the right time. You are ready for this. It is a remarkable feeling when you realize you are truly getting to know yourself better than you ever thought possible.

Set your mood.

Write your intention down in your journal. For this meditation you will be working with emotional healing. If you know the specific area you are going to work on, include that in your intention. If you are exploring to find buried issues, make that part of your intention statement. You should work on the areas you know first.

Complete your pre-meditation breathing exercise.

Script

Journey back to your sacred space.
Let the feeling of peace and awareness wash over you.
Allow all tension to fall away.
Reach out with your heart and mind to find the
bliss and contentment held here in this space for you.
Open your awareness to everything around you.
Spend a moment immersed in the pleasure
of the connection you feel with the universe.
Feel the energy around you.
Allow it to flow through you.
When you are ready, call upon the deity or
guide you wish to work with.
When they arrive, feel their energy stream
around you and breeze through you.

Enjoy their presence.
Send your energy out to combine
with theirs in your sacred space.
Revel in the pleasure of their presence.
When you are ready, think back to a
person or situation that caused you pain.
You may choose a moment or ask your guide to show you.
Replay what happened in your mind.
Watch the event from other points of view.
Watch it from the point of view of others who were there.
Watch it from the viewpoint of your guide.
How could you have handled the situation differently?
How could the others involved have
handled the situation differently?
Know that you can only control your actions.
Was harm to you intentional?
Is the situation forgivable?
What would you like the other person or people to know?
What would you tell them today if you could?
Know that everyone comes into our lives for a reason.
What did you learn from your experience in this situation?
They have taught you a lesson to keep with you.
It may be a positive lesson, or it may be negative—
it might teach you what you do not want to do.
Absolve yourself from blame for how other people
treat you. But learn not to allow it anymore.
Even if you can't forgive the person involved,
it is okay to move on.
Feel that part of your life healing.
It no longer holds power over you.
Your heart is more complete.

You are more complete.
Feel yourself stronger, more in tune with the
universe, more at peace with yourself.
Spend as much time here as you desire.
When you are ready, thank your deity for
their presence, for their love, for their aid.
Bid them farewell.

As of late, this has been my favorite meditation to work through, and it has opened my stubborn eyes many times over. Even when we think we are "fine," cannabis can help show us where we need changes in our lives, where we have been wrong in the past, how we can improve in the future. But over the years, I have had a hard time letting go of certain aspects of my life and certain people. Working through this meditation several times over has helped me to say good-bye when needed.

The nature of cannabis, particularly in a peak experience, allows us to see ourselves and our situations in a true light, not just how we think they are. It takes off our blinders and opens our eyes. It can be a scary prospect, but in the end it brings us a peace we couldn't find otherwise. Seeing yourself without your own preconceived notions of who you are can be a jolting experience. Each time you perform this meditation, you may learn something new about yourself.

At first, this may seem rather daunting. There may be things about yourself that you do not want to know, but the path to enlightenment requires us to look deep inside to heal our emotional selves in order to truly move on. As you complete this meditation, you'll discover that the more you learn the more you want to learn, allowing subsequent sessions to feel more about healing and less about finding your faults.

Meditation 9
JOY: MEETING YOUR
NEEDS FOR THE FUTURE

While the first meditation we did had you deal with looking to the past to find joy in your life, this meditation is designed to connect you with joy in the present and to incorporate joy into your future. We make a decision every single day whether to be happy or not; even with everything life may throw at us, ultimately the choice is still ours. Some days choosing joy is far more difficult than other days. The key is to add at least a little bit of joy to our lives every single day. Life is short; we should be enjoying it to the fullest, yet we often get caught up in the day-to-day rat race, politics, and other negative aspects that suck the joy and happiness right out of our lives. I'm not saying we should stop caring about those other things—not at all—but we do need to counteract the negativity that we get pounded with daily. The joy should outweigh the negativity, massively. When it doesn't, we do not function at our best. While we do need balance in our lives, that doesn't mean things like negativity need to take up half of our time! That much negativity leads to issues in other aspects of our lives. We need the joy in order to be able to pull ourselves through the negative times.

Pure joy is more than just being happy. Pure joy is what you feel deep down inside. It's the awe that overtakes you when looking at the stars and realizing how lucky you are. It's the light in a child's eyes when they experience something they love for the very first time.

We all feel joy to some extent, but what causes it for each of us may be entirely different. Some find joy in serving others, in giving self-lessly. Some find it in the thrill of adventure—the joy of feeling carefree and expecting the unexpected. Some find joy in teaching and sharing with others.

Joy is what can keep us going when times are rough—the remembrances of joy of the past and the prospect of joy in the future. These times, when it is hard to remember or to even fathom the possibility of having joy in the future, we need to remind ourselves this is a falsehood attacking us. Joy is always possible.

This meditation helps you investigate what it is that brings you the greatest joy, and why.

Set your mood.

Write your intention down in your journal. For this meditation you will be looking at what needs must be met for you to experience joy.

Complete your pre-meditation breathing exercise.

Script

Journey back to your sacred space.
Let the feeling of peace and awareness wash over you.
Allow all tension to fall away.
Reach out with your heart and mind to find the bliss
and contentment held here in this space for you.
Open your awareness to everything around you.
Spend a moment immersed in the pleasure of
the connection you feel with the universe.
Feel the energy around you.
Allow it to flow through you.
When you are ready, call upon the deity
or guide you wish to work with.
When they arrive, feel their energy stream
around you and breeze through you.
Enjoy their presence.

Send your energy out to combine
with theirs in your sacred space.
Revel in the pleasure of their presence.
Go back to one of the moments in time that you were
happiest, or allow your guide to show you one.
Relive the moment from your point of view when it occurred.
Think about how it made you feel.
What need did it fulfill for you?
Do you still feel that need is met?
Go to another time of great joy in your life.
Think about how it made you feel.
What need did it fulfill for you?
Do you still feel that need is met?
Visit several more events.
Is there a common theme?
Is there a common need that was met?
Do you still feel the same joy when that need is met?
Turn your mind's eye now to the future.
See yourself five years from now.
See yourself as if anything is possible,
the greatest joys are yours to have.
Where you live, what you do is all up to you.
What does this future look like?
What needs are being met in your ideal
future that are not being met today?
Spend as much time here as you need to
explore these questions and their answers.
When you are ready, thank your deity for
their presence, for their love, for their aid.
Bid them farewell.

End your session by journaling about the questions you answered in this meditation. Use those answers to brainstorm ways you can begin meeting those needs now. How can you bring your reality closer to your ideal future?

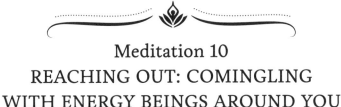

Meditation 10
REACHING OUT: COMINGLING
WITH ENERGY BEINGS AROUND YOU

This meditation is going to help you more later on when you are doing group work, since it is a precursor to help you pick up on the energies of other people and situations around you. Physically, this is an interesting meditation to do in different locations, particularly in a natural environment. It will help you connect with the flora and fauna of a location. You can feel the energies of the trees, flowers, birds, animals, elemental spirits, and more, just by engaging with this meditation. You will find completely different energies in a forest than you would find in a prairie or at a beach. Because of the different environments and different energies, this can be a very fun meditation; keep it light-hearted and upbeat and commune only with positive energies. If you feel an abundance of negative energies at your location, end the meditation and move on to a different location.

Set your mood.

Write your intention down in your journal. For this meditation you will be exploring the energies of your environment.

Complete your pre-meditation breathing exercise.

Script

Journey back to your sacred space.
Let the feeling of peace and awareness wash over you.
Allow all tension to fall away.
Reach out with your heart and mind to find the bliss
and contentment held here in this space for you.
Open your awareness to everything around you.
Spend a moment immersed in the pleasure
of the connection you feel with the universe.
Feel the energy around you.
Allow it to flow through you.
When you are ready, call upon the deity or
guide you wish to work with.
When they arrive, feel their energy stream
around you and breeze through you.
Enjoy their presence.
Send your energy out to combine
with theirs in your sacred space.
Allow your energies to recharge one another.
Revel in the pleasure of their presence.
When you are ready, open your mind's eye
to the area surrounding you.
Enlarge your safe space, allowing in only
the energies you want to join you.
Compare the appearance of each distinct
energy to its physical form.
How do these energies feel as they
pass through and around you?
Spend time interacting with the different
energies, mingling your energy with theirs.

Open your sacred space as wide as you are comfortable,
allowing more energies to come in.
Reach out to each one in an introduction.
Spend as much time as you like here.
Before you close down your space, thank your guide
and all of the energies you encountered for being
present, and for exchanging their energies with you.

End your session by journaling about the different energies, trying to give as much detail as possible. If you'd like, take a canvas or paper and paint or color an image from your meditation. This can serve as a reminder of your connection with the universe. It can also work as a focal point in other meditations.

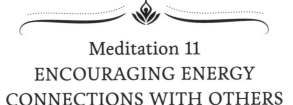

Meditation 11
ENCOURAGING ENERGY
CONNECTIONS WITH OTHERS

While you probably found the idea of the last meditation comforting—feeling your energetic place in nature can be a very welcoming experience—this one may be a little more difficult. Nature can be easy to connect with. Trees and flowers don't tend to have negative energies, but people can. Even if we don't pick up any negative vibes from someone, it can still be difficult to open up to others. This meditation allows you to practice that, in your own sacred space with your guide.

Set your mood.

Write your intention down in your journal. For this meditation you will be exploring your connections with others.

Complete your pre-meditation breathing exercise.

Script

Journey back to your sacred space.
Let the feeling of peace and awareness wash over you.
Allow all tension to fall away.
Reach out with your heart and mind to find the bliss
and contentment held here in this space for you.
Open your awareness to everything around you.
Spend a moment immersed in the pleasure of
the connection you feel with the universe.
Feel the energy around you.
Allow it to flow through you.
When you are ready, call upon the deity or
guide you wish to work with.
When they arrive, feel their energy stream
around you and breeze through you.
Enjoy their presence.
Send your energy out to combine
with theirs in your sacred space.
Revel in the pleasure of their presence.
When you are ready, reach out with your mind's eye to some-
one you care for and love very much.
Feel their spirit mingle with yours, and
invite them to your sacred space.
They may not be physically present, but a
piece of their spirit is here with you.
Mix your energy with theirs in a greeting.
How do you feel when your energies comingle?
Enjoy this experience for a while
and then allow their spirit to go.

Reach out again to someone you know; someone
that you are close to, but not as "attached" to.
Bring their spirit into your sacred space.
Feel the difference between their energy and the previous one.
How does your energy respond?
Share your strength with them, and then pull back again.
Feel how you can control what you share.
You can also control what you receive.
Shut yourself off from receiving their
energy, but allow them to stay.
Practice turning on and off the flow of energy.
When you are done, send their spirit back.
Call the first spirit back.
This spirit you can feel much more intensely
due to your emotional connection.
Practice turning off and on the flow of energy
between you and this spirit.
Spend as much time as you like here.
Before you close down your space, thank
your guide and the spirits you worked with.

Finish your session by journaling about the experience.

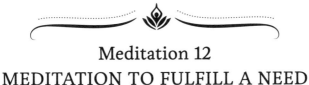

Meditation 12
MEDITATION TO FULFILL A NEED

This is the last meditation you will need to do before being ready to move on to group work. Group work does not mean you need to eliminate your solitary work—not at all! You can go back and perform any of the solitary meditations any time you want.

This last one is going to give you a template to use for meditating for fulfilling a need. You are using your intuition and gathered energy through meditation to effect a change. Through the use of cannabis, you are able to include your deity or guide and all the other energies you have previously encountered and called upon to help effect the change you want to make. While you can do that without cannabis, the intensity and effect is much stronger and more potent with it.

You can also add other spell aspects, such as timing with the full moon, colors, incense, or herbs that relate to your intention.

Set your mood.

Write your intention down in your journal. For this meditation *you* will decide what your intention is.

Complete your pre-meditation breathing exercise.

Script

Journey back to your sacred space.
Let the feeling of peace and awareness wash over you.
Allow all tension to fall away.
Reach out with your heart and mind to find the bliss
and contentment held here in this space for you.
Open your awareness to everything around you.
Spend a moment immersed in the pleasure of
the connection you feel with the universe.
Feel the energy around you.
Allow it to flow through you.
When you are ready, call upon the deity or
guide you wish to work with.
When they arrive, feel their energy stream
around you and breeze through you.

Enjoy their presence.
Send your energy out to combine
with theirs in your sacred space.
Revel in the pleasure of their presence.
Open your sacred space to any other
energies you wish to work with.
Bid them to join with you.
When you are ready, send your intention and
request into your sacred space, sharing it with your
guide and the energies you have invited in.
With your mind's eye, show them the current situation.
Show them how your intent will change the situation.
Listen to your guides and the energies for any feedback.
They may have suggestions for you.
If your guides and energies don't want to
proceed, don't force the matter.
Take the feedback to weigh and
then return at a different time.
When you have reached a consensus, you will know.
Focus on building energy all around
your intent, your desired outcome.
See and feel it in front of you and all
around you in your sacred space.
Spend as much time here as you need.
Watch and feel as the energy around you builds.
When you are ready, set it off into the universe—as if your
sacred space suddenly, yet safely,
explodes out into the universe.
You are still safe in your sacred space, but the
energy shoots through the barrier, dispensing
where it is needed to effect the desired change.

Allow your energy to return to a normal level.
Spend a few moments grounding your mind and emotions.
Bring yourself back to your bliss-filled state.
When you are ready, thank your deity or guide
for their presence, for their love, for their aid.
Bid them farewell.

Journal about the experience of this meditation.

You've now learned a specific format to perform your meditations, and if you wish to continue to follow the format, do so. But now that you are no longer a beginner, feel free to start experimenting with writing your own or performing "free thought" meditations.

You now have the necessary skills to move on to group work. Keep up your solitary practice and begin building your own meditations for your own needs. Moving on to group work can be a life-changing, society-altering experience. Cannabis can build bonds.

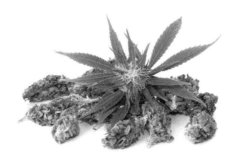

Chapter 6

Creating a Group Practice

Working with a group can be an incredibly deep and powerful experience. While spiritually rewarding, it's also a lot of fun. Pagan groups combine their talents together to help other people or the environment, or to enact social change through rituals, spells, or other energy work. Your group can do the same through cannabis-aided meditation.

You've already learned how to work on your own inner issues. Within a group, you will work with others to focus your energies outward on external issues.

Finding a group may be the most difficult part of your journey, or you may already know plenty of people who are wanting to do the same thing. The key is communication. Let others know what you are looking for. Social media is always the first option these days, but you can also contact your local metaphysical stores, head shops, and cannabis dispensaries. How difficult it is to find other like-minded individuals may be very dependent on what the law allows in your area. goddess knows I can't wait for the day that nature wins.

You may already have your second group member: your partner. If your partner is someone you have been able to take turns and fully share this experience with, then they should also be ready to move from working as a partner to working as a group member. You won't need each other in the same ways any longer, as by now you should be comfortable and confident in your dosing and meditations.

Instead of a partner, groups should be led by a "leader" or "host." I prefer the term *host*, as it doesn't imply anyone is in charge of anyone else. Your host is there to guide you through the meditations and to help ensure comfort and deal with any issues should they arise. Your host is sober for the event, catering to the needs of each guest. All participants should take turns at being host for a session.

The host is also responsible for setting the timing for the meditation. If the group plans to work for an hour, then the host must know how to read the meditation to stretch it out over an hour. In the first few meditations, the host will want to remember to speak slowly, allowing for plenty of time between each statement. As you build this foundation and develop more practice at calling in the space and deities, the host can leave less time in between statements. For example, for meditation one, you may leave two to three minutes between each statement, but by the time the group has advanced to meditation five, you may cut that time down to a minute, and by meditation ten, maybe down to thirty seconds. It is important that the group communicates about how much time they need to be comfortable. You should always decide how much time to allow for workings ahead of time, so the host and participants can be properly prepared. Participants need timing information to know what kind of dosing they will need to maintain. I can't emphasize enough how convenient an oil or concentrate vape pen can be in doing meditation work. No need for lighters or refills; it's just inhale and go. It helps keep the mood going due to its minimal disruption.

Before any workings take place, there will be decisions to be made and rules to set. This should be done at your first meetup (cannabis free).

Depending on where you live, weed can be expensive. I hear it's far cheaper in California than it is here in Illinois—which I'm also told is currently the most expensive state. How will your group deal with expenses? If you are lucky enough to be able to grow, that helps—quite a bit actually! Otherwise, cost is something your group needs to discuss. I recommend everyone is responsible for their own stash. Perhaps a collection can be taken at each meeting to pay for refreshments for the next meeting, or volunteers can be assigned to make and bring refreshments. Go with whatever system works best for your members. Refreshments can be both "normal" and cannabis-infused to use throughout the meditation to help keep people in the proper mindset, or even to start the evening off. I have included a section in this book with an introduction to cooking with cannabis, along with recipes perfect for group settings.

You will need to decide where you will practice. It may always be the same location, or it may be several different locations, dependent upon who is hosting. Even if you meet at the same location all the time, you will still switch hosting responsibilities. Your group can meet indoors or outdoors, following the same guidelines as your individual work. Be sure your location is comfortable, safe, and legal. Participants may want to provide their own cushions, pillows, blankets, or other items to ensure comfort.

Each member should also bring something to each session as a representation. For example, when calling to the Divine Feminine, each member should bring a representation of the Divine Feminine. Everyone needs to remember that this group is very much about participation. Besides, the more you put into it, the more you will get out of it. You want everyone's energy to be represented.

How often will you meet? I recommend at least monthly. You can build this practice as much as you want or keep it smaller and more casual. It's always about what works for you. It will also depend on what you are working on. You may eventually want to plan special meditations for full or new moons to work on specific goals or energy work. Your group decides what the group's needs are. You may even want to give your group a name. Make it what you all want and need it to be. Be conscious of each other's needs and find solutions and compromises to work for everyone.

The first few times your group meets, you need to spend time getting to know each other and learning how you mesh. Basically, you need to hang out and get stoned. Combining people to work together means you all must learn how to hit your high or peak experience in tandem, or at the very least, as close as you can muster. Therefore, your first group sessions should be centered on finding out how to best do that. All the participants should know what it takes to achieve their own peak. Those that hit a peak first will need to sustain theirs long enough for others to "catch up," or they should start their dosing later. These dry runs give you and the rest of the group information you can use to help sync everyone one up to work in conjunction later. The first three meetups shouldn't contain a meditation at all. First get to know each other, set your rules and guidelines, select your location, hosts, food, and money plan—basically, discuss all the things. The second and third time you meet, get stoned. Now, that doesn't sound too difficult, does it? You can spend some time at each of these events to practice your deep breathing together.

By the fourth time you meet, you will be ready to enjoy some cannabis-infused edibles and this new leg of your journey.

When you are ready to begin your practice, it will proceed very much the same as your solitary practice. Set the mood with incense, lighting, and music. Representations or other items brought by members should be placed on an altar in the center of your space. (Your group may add any other altar items you agree upon.)

Write your intention down in your journal. When you begin group practice, you may no longer see a need for keeping track of dosing information. If you want to continue to record dosing information, please feel free, but at this point you are far past that being the most important piece of information. You may still want to keep track of the strain, though, if you are still experimenting with different ones (and with all the different ones out there and new ones being cultivated all the time, you can experiment with strains for a lifetime).

Finally, get comfy and dose away!

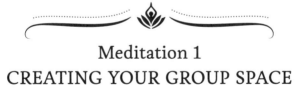

Meditation 1
CREATING YOUR GROUP SPACE

Each group member already has their own personal sacred space. Now you must learn how to merge them together. You will use the skills you learned in the "Reaching Out" meditation to join together with your mates in the spiritual realm.

Set your mood.

Record your intention in your journal—you may want to use both a personal journal and a group journal. This is another decision you will need to make. A group journal can have the host making all entries, or you can work out how your group wants to handle it.

Complete your pre-meditation breathing exercise.

Script

Journey back to your own sacred space.
Let the feeling of peace and awareness wash over you.
Allow all tension to fall away.
Reach out with your heart and mind to find the bliss
and contentment held here in this space for you.
Open your awareness to everything around you.
Spend a moment immersed in the pleasure of
the connection you feel with the universe.
Feel the energy around you.
Allow it to flow through you.
Still in your place, reach out to the others here.
Feel their presence.
See their energy.
Their place mingles with yours.
You blend and merge, interlacing together.
This space is our space.
We are all here.
We are all one.
Spend as much time here as you need.
When ready, bid farewell to the energies of
each other and return to your own sacred space.

Finish the session with time for journaling.

I highly recommend performing this meditation together several times before moving on. There is no rush to get to the end of the book. Enjoy your time with one another. Learn each other's energies. Experience the intimacy the joined sacred space creates. You can also make this meditation as short or as long as you like, but decide beforehand so that everyone can maintain their peak without interruption for the duration of the session. We will use this meditation as a base to build upon.

Meditation 2
CONNECTING TO THE DIVINE FEMININE

Yes, this is going to be just as incredible as it sounds. This time, after you all come together in Spirit, you will each invite your own representation of the Divine Feminine, whatever that is for you, to join you in the group. The only other requirement is that this entity be one you have worked with before, preferably several times. Don't use group work for outside exploration; work with what you know and experiment in your solitary practice.

Set your mood.

Record your intention in your journal.

Complete your pre-meditation breathing exercise.

Script

> *Journey back to your own sacred space.*
> *Let the feeling of peace and awareness wash over you.*
> *Allow all tension to fall away.*
> *Reach out with your heart and mind to find the bliss*
> *and contentment held here in this space for you.*
> *Open your awareness to everything around you.*

Spend a moment immersed in the pleasure
of the connection you feel with the universe.
Feel the energy around you.
Allow it to flow through you.
Still in your place, reach out to the others here.
Feel their presence.
See their energy.
Their place interlaces with yours.
You blend and merge, interlacing together.
This space is our space.
We are all here.
We are all one.
We are all one.

Allow several minutes to elapse.

Return to yourself again.
Separate but still connected.
Feel your strength.
With your mind's eye, call out to your goddess, to your guide.
Ask her to join by your side.
Welcome her into the shared sacred space.
As she joins, recognize her energy.
Allow the other energies, the other entities, around you
to fade softly, allowing hers to become dominant.
Reach out and connect with her through your mind's eye.
Send your energy to intermingle with hers.
Your energies swirl around and through each other.

Allow several minutes here.

Slowly open your mind's eye to the energies
around you, the ones faded to the background.
Allow them to rise to full power
again within your visualization.
They are all joined by their own
representation of the Divine Feminine.
Take turns introducing your deities;
this may be done silently or out loud.
Spend time in the presence of divinity.
Learn the energies each sends to you.
Spend as much time here as you need.
When ready, bid farewell to the deities of the
others; allow them to fade from your mind's eye.
Bid farewell to your deity; thank her for attending.
Bid farewell to the energies of each other
and return to your own sacred space.

Finish the session with time for journaling.

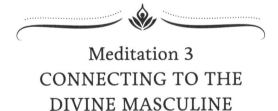

Meditation 3
CONNECTING TO THE
DIVINE MASCULINE

The script for this meditation will be the same as for the Divine Feminine, substituting male gendered pronouns where appropriate. The reasons for it being the same script are practical ones. Repetition is a good way to learn. Learning the words and order of a meditation makes it easier to perform the meditation. You know what to expect and what work you need to do. Also, whenever we call in deities to our group work, it can be done the same way, allowing the user to determine which deity to call in. Because we use each meditation as a base for the next (in the beginning ones), this is imperative to keep the flow going. Those who wish to work with a god may, and those wishing to work with a goddess may also do so all at the same time.

Set your mood.

Record your intention in your journal.

Complete your pre-meditation breathing exercise.

Script

Journey back to your own sacred space.
Let the feeling of peace and awareness wash over you.
Allow all tension to fall away.
Reach out with your heart and mind to find the bliss
and contentment held here in this space for you.
Open your awareness to everything around you.
Spend a moment immersed in the pleasure
of the connection you feel with the universe.
Feel the energy around you.
Allow it to flow through you.
Still in your place, reach out to the others here.
Feel their presence.
See their energy.
Their place mingles with yours.
You blend and merge, interlacing together.
This space is our space.
We are all here.
We are all one.
We are all one.

Allow several minutes to elapse.

Return to yourself again.
Separate but still connected.
Feel your strength.
With your mind's eye, call out to your god, to your guide.
Ask him to join by your side.
Welcome him into the shared sacred space.
As he joins, recognize his energy.
Allow the other energies, the other entities around you,
to fade softly, allowing his to become dominant.
Reach out and connect with him through your mind's eye.
Send your energy to intermingle with his.
Your energies swirl around and through each other.

The host should allow several minutes here.

Slowly open your mind's eye to the energies
around you, the ones faded to the background.
Allow them to rise to full power again in your visualization.
They are all joined by their own
representation of the Divine Masculine.
Take turns introducing your deities;
this may be done silently or out loud.
Spend time in the presence of divinity.
Learn the energies each sends to you.
Spend as much time here as you need.
When ready, bid farewell to the deities of the
others; allow them to fade from your mind's eye.
Bid farewell to your deity; thank him for attending.
Bid farewell to the energies of each other
and return to your own sacred space.

Finish the session with time for journaling.

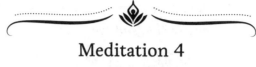

Meditation 4
TRUST TRANCE DANCE

Trust between members is one of the most important aspects of a successful group working. If you do not feel you can trust your fellow group members, it makes it very difficult to give 100 percent of yourself in workings with them.

This meditation is designed to help build trust between group members using the aids of meditation, cannabis, intimacy, and music. You may choose a different soundtrack if you like, but I love the album *Gratitude Joy* by Anand Anugrah and Paul Avgerinos for this meditation.

This meditation will be different than what you have done before. While the beginning will take place in your normal meditative pose, whether this be seated or lying down, you will later get up for some trance dance work. You will need to make sure you have room for this to occur. This will be a slow, rhythmic trance dance, not fast or energy building. While movement can be far more difficult for some people than it is for others, do not let that hold you back. Sitting in a chair and slowly moving your head, neck, and shoulders, or perhaps moving your hands to the rhythm are all completely acceptable ways to participate. It's more about energy flowing than your actual physical movements. Use your mind and visualize the energy moving around you, flowing through yourself and your group members.

Slow dancing has a certain intimacy to it. Remember that intimacy and sexuality are not the same thing. This exercise is not about sexual arousal; it is about experiencing shared energy, which is its own particular kind of energy. It gives you a bond with your group members. If you have a certain strain that you associate the word *groovy* with, that's the strain you want to use for this meditation. Decide beforehand how much time you want to spend in the trance dance part of this meditation. Five minutes or ten minutes or more—it's up to you and up to the host to guide the participants. This is a meditation your group may want to perform several times, and you can do so, increasing the amount of time in the trance dance for each session.

Set your mood.

Record your intention in your journal.

Complete your pre-meditation breathing exercise.

Script

Journey back to your own sacred space.
Let the feeling of peace and awareness wash over you.
Allow all tension to fall away.
Reach out with your heart and mind to find the bliss
and contentment held here in this space for you.
Open your awareness to everything around you.
Spend a moment immersed in the pleasure
of the connection you feel with the universe.
Feel the energy around you.
Allow it to flow through you.
Still in your place, reach out to the others here.
Feel their presence.
See their energy.
Their place mingles with yours.
You blend and merge, interlacing together.
This space is our space.
We are all here.
We are all one.
We are all one.

Allow several minutes to elapse.

Return to yourself again.
Separate but still connected.
Feel your strength.
With your mind's eye, call out to your deity, to your guide.
Ask them to join by your side.
Welcome them into the shared sacred space.
As they join, recognize their energy.
Allow the other energies and other entities around you to fade
softly, allowing your guide's energy to become dominant.
Reach out and connect with them through your mind's eye.
Send your energy to intermingle with theirs.
Your energies swirl around and through each other.

Allow several minutes here.

Slowly open your mind's eye to the energies
around you, the ones faded to the background.
Allow them to rise to full power again in your visualization.
They are all joined by their own representation of divinity.
Spend time in the presence of divinity.
When you are ready, rise to standing.
Be aware of your surroundings, closing your eyes
but opening them again whenever you want to.
Feel the music flowing through you.
Begin rocking your body left to right.
Feel your shoulders push and pull you in
each direction, back and forth.
Rhythmically.

Allow your hips to pick up the rhythm.
Let either your shoulders or hips lead the
dance through the infinity symbol.
Lift to the right, drop, lift to the left, drop.
Draw it out.
Be mindful of the energy you send out,
and the energy you receive.
Fill your heart with love and trust.
Send this to each other.
Feel the trust and love you are receiving.

The host will need to keep track of the time.

Slow down your movements.
Slower.
Slower.
Feel your energy return to you, refreshed.
Return to your seated position.
Hold the energy close to you; allow
it to soak back into you slowly.
Spend as much time here as needed.
When ready, bid farewell to the deities of
the others; allow them to fade from your mind's eye.
Bid farewell to your deity; thank them for attending.
Bid farewell to the energies of each other
and return to your own sacred space.

Finish the session with time for journaling.

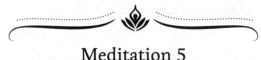

Meditation 5
HEALING A DISTANT SOUL

In your solitary work, you learned how to perform meditations to heal yourself both physically and emotionally. Now you will combine your energies with other people to send out distance healing to someone who is not physically present with you. You do not need to know what specific healing they need, but it does help. This meditation can be used whether the healing is needed physically or emotionally, and by human or by animal.

Set your mood.

Record your intention in your journal.

Complete your pre-meditation breathing exercise.

Script

Journey back to your own sacred space.
Let the feeling of peace and awareness wash over you.
Allow all tension to fall away.
Reach out with your heart and mind to find the bliss
and contentment held here in this space for you.
Open your awareness to everything around you.
Spend a moment immersed in the pleasure
of the connection you feel with the universe.
Feel the energy around you.
Allow it to flow through you.
Still in your place, reach out to the others here.
Feel their presence.
See their energy.
Their place mingles with yours.

You blend and merge, interlacing together.
This space is our space.
We are all here.
We are all one.
We are all one.

Allow several minutes to elapse.

Return to yourself again.
Separate but still connected.
Feel your strength.
With your mind's eye, call out to your deity, to your guide.
Ask them to join by your side.
Welcome them into the shared sacred space.
As they join, recognize their energy.
Allow the other energies and other entities around you
to fade softly, allowing theirs to become dominant.
Reach out and connect with them through your mind's eye.
Send your energy to intermingle with theirs.
Your energies swirl around and through each other.

Allow several minutes here.

Slowly open your mind's eye to the energies
around you, the ones faded to the background.
Allow them to rise to full power again in your visualization.
They are all joined by their own representation of divinity.
Spend time in the presence of divinity.

Allow several minutes here.

Focus your mind now to (host names the recipient
and gives any other information known—for example,
"Brian, who needs healing for his broken left arm.").
Reach out to find his energy. (Use the appropriate
pronoun—for our example Brian goes by he/him/his.)
Search for him; you will know him when you find him.
Find his energy reaching out for help.
Surround his energy with yours, not smothering but gentle.
Gently pillowing, comforting.
Where his energy is darkened, shower it
with white light energy from your own.
Wash away the dull.
Wash away the pain.
Leave only whole, clean, white light.
It radiates for a time, then slowly blends in
to the rest of his energy field.
Changing colors until it fits, perfectly new.
Perfectly healed.
Allow his spirit to return to where it was,
as you pull your energy back home to you.
Feel your energy return to you, refreshed.
Renewed.
Hold the energy close to you; allow
it to soak back into you slowly.
Spend as much time here as needed.
When ready, bid farewell to the deities of the
others; allow them to fade from your mind's eye.
Bid farewell to your deity; thank them for attending.
Bid farewell to the energies of each other
and return to your own sacred space.

Finish the session with time for journaling.

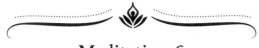

Meditation 6
PROTECTION DURING A NATURAL DISASTER

While "thoughts & prayers" has become a national joke, let's not confuse the lack of compassion and empathy in politics with the true compassion and empathy of the rest of the world. When there is a major hurricane, earthquake, tsunami, wildfire, tornado, or other natural disaster somewhere in the world, there is really not a whole lot many of us can do at that exact moment. Some can donate money, but we can't teleport there to help. We can't use superpowers to make the event stop. We can't turn back time and prevent it from happening in the first place.

But we can send our energy and ask our deities to do to the same at our sides, to help protect the people who are in harm's way. This can be deeply emotional for people, so be supportive of one another during this experience.

Set your mood.

Record your intention in your journal.

Complete your pre-meditation breathing exercise.

Script

Journey back to your own sacred space.
Let the feeling of peace and awareness wash over you.
Allow all tension to fall away.
Reach out with your heart and mind to find the bliss
and contentment held here in this space for you.
Open your awareness to everything around you.
Spend a moment immersed in the pleasure
of the connection you feel with the universe.
Feel the energy around you.

Allow it to flow through you.
Still in your place, reach out to the others here.
Feel their presence.
See their energy.
Their place mingles with yours.
You blend and merge, interlacing together.
This space is our space.
We are all here.
We are all one.
We are all one.

Allow several minutes to elapse.

Return to yourself again.
Separate but still connected.
Feel your strength.
With your mind's eye, call out to your deity, to your guide.
Ask them to join you by your side.
Welcome them into the shared sacred space.
As they join, recognize their energy.
Allow the other energies and other entities around you
to fade softly, allowing theirs to become dominant.
Reach out and connect with them through your mind's eye.
Send your energy to intermingle with theirs.
Your energies swirl around and through each other.

Allow several minutes here.

Slowly open your mind's eye to the energies
around you, the ones faded to the background.
Allow them to rise to full power again in your visualization.
They are all joined by their own representation of divinity.

Turn your mind now to the task at hand.
Your energy is strong and powerful.
Right now, it's needed elsewhere.
By other people.
The people need it.
The animals need it.
The land needs it.
Using your mind's eye, find the location.
See what is happening.
See the people.
See the animals.
See the land.
Send a protective energy out over them.
Feel them being held in a strong,
safe embrace of positive energy.
Ask your deities to lend their aid, to watch over, to protect.
Swaddle their energy, holding it close to you, protectively.
You feel the rage at your back, but must push back against it.
See the (event) weakening, losing power, ending, dying.
Allow it to pass from your mind; it's gone and done.
Envision the area, the people, the animals, the land, all healing.
Coming back to life.
Watch as it recovers, not the same as before, but still beautiful.
The loss will not be forgotten.
You will leave behind a piece of your energy.
Energy to build a shield.
Send a portion of your energy out to the area; there it
will join with the others to form a dome of protection.
See the energies combine together, forming
a dome, surrounding, protecting, providing.

When you are sure the dome is intact and in
place, say your goodbye to this place.
Bring your energy back to the sacred space.
Allow your energies to intermingle once again.
Comfort and cleanse one another's energies.
Feel the rest of your energy return to you, refreshed.
Renewed.
Hold the energy close to you, allow
it to soak back into you slowly.
Spend as much time here as needed.
When ready, bid farewell to the deities of the others,
allow them to fade from your mind's eye.
Bid farewell to your deity, thank them for attending.
Bid farewell to the energies of each other
and return to your own sacred space.

Finish the session with time for journaling.

When you are finished with this meditation, you may have a strong desire to do something, anything, to help the people in the affected area. DO IT. No amount of help is too small. You have a group of people you are working with—combine your resources, talents, skills, and connections and see what you can come up with. In a situation where a person has literally nothing left but their life, no amount of assistance is too small.

We must be the change we so desperately need in the world.

Meditation 7
HEALING PLANET EARTH

Whether you see earth as a planet or as the Mother Gaia, we should all be concerned for her welfare. I was recently disheartened to see a conversation in the Chicago Pagans Facebook group where it was made quite clear, out of those members who took the time to respond, that many of them did not believe the science claiming we are very close to the point of no return for sustaining human life on earth. Worse still was the number who didn't really seem to care, saying that even if it is true, they will be gone then anyway.

I don't know where these attitudes came from, but they are literally the opposite of what many Pagans claim to believe. Whether you believe the science or not, if the end outcome is the destruction of all life, why wouldn't you want to err on the side of caution? It's not like we are killing off only mosquitos; it's everything. Maybe it's time we start taking it a bit more seriously.

If you practice an earth-based religion, why wouldn't you want the earth to be happy and healthy, and here?

I believe, and really hope it's true, that there are far more Pagans out there in the world who do have a strong connection with the earth and understand that not only do we owe our survival to her, but we owe her survival to our children and grandchildren and ancestors down the line. She has supported us for thousands of years and we need to support her back, sending energy to help her. We are her caretakers, and right now we are failing.

Set your mood.

Record your intention in your journal.

Complete your pre-meditation breathing exercise.

Script

Journey back to your own sacred space.
Let the feeling of peace and awareness wash over you.
Allow all tension to fall away.
Reach out with your heart and mind to find the bliss
and contentment held here in this space for you.
Open your awareness to everything around you.
Spend a moment immersed in the pleasure
of the connection you feel with the universe.
Feel the energy around you.
Allow it to flow through you.
Still in your place, reach out to the others here.
Feel their presence.
See their energy.
Their place mingles with yours.
You blend and merge, interlacing together.
This space is our space.
We are all here.
We are all one.
We are all one.

Allow several minutes to elapse.

Return to yourself again.
Separate but still connected.
Feel your strength.
With your mind's eye, call out to your deity, to your guide.
Ask them to join you by your side.
Welcome them into the shared sacred space.
As they join, recognize their energy.

Allow the other energies, the other entities around you,
to fade softly, allowing theirs to become dominant.
Reach out and connect with them through your mind's eye.
Send your energy to intermingle with theirs.
Your energies swirl around and through each other.

The host should allow several minutes here.

Slowly open your mind's eye to the energies
around you, the ones faded to the background.
Allow them to rise to full power again in your visualization.
They are all joined by their own representation of divinity.
Turn your mind now to the task at hand.
Visualize the earth in whatever aspect you prefer to see her.
The blue, green, white, round planet.
The pregnant belly of Gaia.
See her beauties.
See her strengths.
See her traumas.
See her weaknesses.
Feel her love.
Feel her pain.
Send your energy where you feel it needed.
Fill in where the earth is damaged or weak.
Lend her the energy she needs to heal.
See and feel your energy repairing her damage.
Building her up.
Clearing her air, her land, her waters.
Visualize her healing. Clean.
Feel the love, protection, and repairing strength of your mates.
Join together to heal her as best you can.

Spend as much time here as you need.
When ready, bid farewell to the deities of the others,
allow them to fade from your mind's eye.
Bid farewell to your deity; thank them for attending.
Bid farewell to the energies of each other
and return to your own sacred space.

Finish the session with time for journaling.

Be sure to practice in the real world what you preach in the spiritual world. How can you help heal the planet? While I don't expect anyone to go completely off the grid or to leave no carbon footprint, there are other, less dramatic things you can do to help. Vote. Vote for the people who want to save the planet. Vote with your dollars for the companies that are being ethically responsible. Do what you can in your own little corner of the world and encourage others to do the same in theirs.

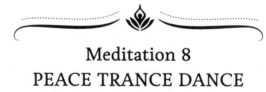

Meditation 8
PEACE TRANCE DANCE

If all our world's conflicts could come to an end with a simple meditation of peace, what a wonderful world this would be. Unfortunately, the real world is nothing like that. We can pray for peace, we can work spells for peace, but until we truly begin to live peace, we will never obtain it.

That doesn't mean we shouldn't try.

I don't know if worldwide peace and harmony is truly possible. But I do know we could have more peace than we do now. We can always have more. In order to have more peace, we must be more peaceful.

While the meditation and process itself here are very similar to what we did when working with trust, our intention is where we will see the difference. This meditation is centered on finding your inner peace and sharing it outward into the universe. It isn't going to solve the world's problems, but it may help you enact change in your local area by sharing peace with others and letting the message flow. Because I love the concept of trance dance, particularly when combined with the lack of inhibition of a peak experience, I wanted to be sure to include a separate opportunity to practice in this manner. You can use the music I previously recommended or if you want, you can "assign" specific songs to specific meditations. Two other songs I enjoy for trance dance work are from David and Steve Gordon. "Four Direction Groove" is off the album *Drum Cargo Rhythms*, and "Dancing for a Vision" is on *Sacred Earth Drums*. Don't be limited by my suggestions! There is so much out there to choose from, and these trance dance meditations can be performed over and over again, so please try them out with different songs.

Set your mood.

Record your intention in your journal.

Complete your pre-meditation breathing exercise.

Script

Journey back to your own sacred space.
Let the feeling of peace and awareness wash over you.
Allow all tension to fall away.
Reach out with your heart and mind to find the bliss
and contentment held here in this space for you.
Open your awareness to everything around you.
Spend a moment immersed in the pleasure
of the connection you feel with the universe.
Feel the energy around you.

Allow it to flow through you.
Still in your place, reach out to the others here.
Feel their presence.
See their energy.
Their place mingles with yours.
You blend and merge, interlacing together.
This space is our space.
We are all here.
We are all one.
We are all one.

Allow several minutes to elapse.

Return to yourself again.
Separate but still connected.
Feel your strength.
With your mind's eye, call out to your deity, to your guide.
Ask them to join by your side.
Welcome them into the shared sacred space.
As they join, recognize their energy.
Allow the other energies, the other entities around
you to fade softly, allowing theirs to become dominate.
Reach out and connect with them through your mind's eye.
Send your energy to intermingle with theirs.
Your energies swirl around and through each other.
Slowly open your mind's eye to the energies
around you, the ones faded to the background.
Allow them to rise to full power again in your visualization.
They are all joined by their own representation of divinity.
Turn your mind now to the task at hand.
When you are ready, rise to standing.

Be aware of your surroundings, closing your eyes
but opening them again whenever you want.
Feel the music flowing through you.
Begin rocking your body left to right to the music.
Feel your shoulders push and pull you in
each direction, back and forth.
Rhythmically.
Encourage your hips to pick up the rhythm.
Let either your shoulders or hips lead the
dance through the infinity symbol.
Lift to the right, drop, lift to the left, drop.
Drawing it out.
Be mindful of the energy you send out,
and the energy you receive.
Feel yourself at peace, at one with the universe.
Find the energy inside you that radiates peace.
Feel it grow, illuminating a pathway through
your body, swirling through your chakras.
Veining off in all directions.
It shoots off of you, spreading through the sacred space.
Absorb the energy coming from the others.
Refresh and recharge your energy with theirs.
As you move, the energy shifts with you.
Feel at one with peace, at one with each
other, at one with the universe.
We are all one. (Repeat as needed.)
Send the energy of peace out of the sacred space.
Watch as it gently rains down upon the earth.
Encompasses and envelopes the earth.
The earth and all her people.
All her inhabitants.
Send peace to all.

The host will need to keep track of the time.

Slow down your movements.
Slower.
Slower.
Feel your energy return to you, refreshed.
Return to your seated position.
Hold the energy close to you;
allow it to soak back into you slowly.
Spend as much time here as needed.
When ready, bid farewell to the deities of the
others; allow them to fade from your mind's eye.
Bid farewell to your deity; thank them for attending.
Bid farewell to the energies of each other
and return to your own sacred space.

Finish the session with time for journaling.

Meditation 9
CONNECTING TO OTHER
GROUPS ON THE SPIRITUAL PLANE

Your group will be limited in physical size because of forces working against it. Not only do you have to find people willing and able, you need to find people to work with that are within a reasonable distance to travel. Legality issues may also affect your group size.

The spiritual plane doesn't have the same limitations. You can send your workings out onto the spiritual plane at the same time as other groups in a coordinated effort. More group efforts have been made lately, and it is wonderful to see support from all around the world coming together. The more we join together, the more we help one another, the better we all become.

Once you learn how to connect with other groups on the spiritual plane, you can perform specific workings simultaneously for added power. The more connections we make, the more healing and helping we can do.

Set your mood.

Record your intention in your journal.

Complete your pre-meditation breathing exercise.

Script

Journey back to your own sacred space.
Let the feeling of peace and awareness wash over you.
Allow all tension to fall away.
Reach out with your heart and mind to find the bliss
and contentment held here in this space for you.
Open your awareness to everything around you.
Spend a moment immersed in the pleasure
of the connection you feel with the universe.
Feel the energy around you.
Allow it to flow through you.
Still in your place, reach out to the others here.
Feel their presence.
See their energy.
Their place mingles with yours.
You blend and merge, interlacing together.
This space is our space.
We are all here.
We are all one.
We are all one.

Allow several minutes to elapse.

Return to yourself again.
Separate but still connected.
Feel your strength.
With your mind's eye, call out to your deity, to your guide.
Ask them to join by your side.
Welcome them into the shared sacred space.
As they join, recognize their energy.
Allow the other energies, the other entities around you
to fade softly, allowing theirs to become dominant.
Reach out and connect with them through your mind's eye.
Send your energy to intermingle with theirs.
Your energies swirl around and through each other.
Slowly open your mind's eye to the energies
around you, the ones faded to the background.
Allow them to rise to full power again in your visualization.
They are all joined by their own representation of divinity.
Turn your mind now to the task at hand.
Send your energies out further than you have before.
Feel them reaching, stretching, like a
starburst through your shared space.
The energy light stretches on for infinity; even when
you can no longer see it with your mind's eye, you
feel it still there, stretching, reaching, detecting.
Waiting to encounter the energy of
another group reaching out to you.
Open your mind, searching for the trails of another group.
When you find a trace, guide your mates to it.
Direct your energy toward theirs,
meeting theirs, magnifying both.

Strengthening the signal to draw in others.
Light radiates outward, like beams from
the sun, breaking through the clouds.
Feel and see their energy coming back to you.
Spend as much time here as you'd like,
sending and receiving energies with other groups.
When ready, bid farewell to the deities of the others;
allow them to fade from your mind's eye.
Bid farewell to your deity; thank them for attending.
Bid farewell to the energies of each other
and return to your own sacred space.

Finish the session with time for journaling.

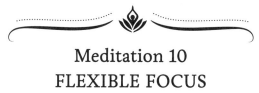

Meditation 10
FLEXIBLE FOCUS

When you have a situation that none of the other meditations fit into, you can use this meditation to focus on the issue at hand. This can be used to help send energy to a specific situation or to help discover solutions to a problem. It is a way to focus the group on a specific issue not previously discussed. This is a multipurpose, generic working you can use in a variety of situations until your group begins writing its own meditations. The format and process will stay the same, only your intent will change with each session. The host will explain the intention more thoroughly during setup and dosing.

Set your mood.

Record your intention in your journal.

Complete your pre-meditation breathing exercise.

Script

Journey back to your own sacred space.
Let the feeling of peace and awareness wash over you.
Allow all tension to fall away.
Reach out with your heart and mind to find the bliss
and contentment held here in this space for you.
Open your awareness to everything around you.
Spend a moment immersed in the pleasure
of the connection you feel with the universe.
Feel the energy around you.
Allow it to flow through you.
Still in your place, reach out to the others here.
Feel their presence.
See their energy.
Their place mingles with yours.
You blend and merge, interlacing together.
This space is our space.
We are all here.
We are all one.
We are all one.

Allow several minutes to elapse.

Return to yourself again.
Separate but still connected.
Feel your strength.
With your mind's eye, call out to your deity, to your guide.
Ask them to join by your side.
Welcome them into the shared sacred space.
As they join, recognize their energy.

Allow the other energies, the other entities around you,
to fade softly, allowing theirs to become dominant.
Reach out and connect with them through your mind's eye.
Send your energy to intermingle with theirs.
Your energies swirl around and through each other.

Allow several minutes here.

Slowly open your mind's eye to the energies
around you, the ones faded to the background.
Allow them to rise to full power again in your visualization.
They are all joined by their own representation of divinity.
Turn your mind now to the task at hand.

Host makes a statement of intention.

Join energy with your group mates.
Focus your mind and your energy on our intent.
Visualize the changes that need to take
place to bring about our intention.

Host may give more details.

Focus your energy on making these changes happen.
We ask our deities to lend their support
and to grant these changes be made.
Continue visualizing the outcome we want to see.
See it in your heart.
See it your mind.
See it in our future.
When ready, bid farewell to the deities of the
others; allow them to fade from your mind's eye.

> *Bid farewell to your deity; thank them for attending.*
> *Bid farewell to the energies of each other*
> *and return to your own sacred space.*

Finish the session with time for journaling.

This meditation can also be done as trance dance if you want to add to the raising of energy.

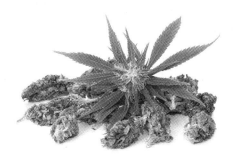

Chapter 7
Cooking with Cannabis

Just the idea of cooking with cannabis may sound daunting, but it really isn't nearly as difficult as it sounds. There are many ways cannabis can be used in recipes, and as I stated earlier in this book, in some places, terpenes are even extracted and can be used to add the specific flavors and qualities each terpene contains.

There are easy ways of adding weed to your menu without having to be a gourmet cannabis chef, just by infusing basic ingredients with cannabis—ingredients such as butter, oil, and alcohol.

Some people love the different flavors and scents that can be combined and created; some hate the taste and smell; and to some it all seems the same anyway. (According to my husband, it all smells like skunk.)

For those of you who are not gourmet chefs and would still like to reap the rewards, this is where you get to learn how.

It's important to remember that smoking and eating are not the same thing. When eating cannabis, the THC will affect you much more strongly than it does when smoking. It will take longer for the high to hit, and the high will last much longer. As with all forms of consumption, remember to go slow. You can always eat more if you need to, but give yourself plenty of time between doses (a good thirty minutes minimum).

Another big hint—if you have enough weed to do so—is to make butters and oils at different strengths or make them as strong as you can. Different strengths are convenient. If you are going to make cookies and need two cups of butter, your cookies will have a much higher potency than something that only uses a small amount of butter. What you can do is make a "normal" dose of seven grams to a cup for things like cookies, which use a lot of butter. Then infuse another batch of butter with fourteen grams to a cup to make it more potent, and use it for recipes where you only use a little butter. If you make it stronger, you can always cut it with noninfused butter or oil. In the cookie example, you could use one cup of strong cannabutter and one cup of regular butter to equal your two cups.

Before we get into recipes, the first topic we need to cover is preparing weed for consumption and how we can put it into different usable forms.

Decarboxylation

To prepare your cannabis to be used in cooking, the first step is to decarboxylate it. Basically, this means you need to heat it up to a particular temperature for a set amount of time, allowing the chemical reaction to take place, and therefore activating the THC and THC-A in the cannabis.

If you know you are going to be cooking cannabis a lot, I highly recommend investing in a decarboxylator. There currently are not too many options available. There are options available online for just over $200.

Why invest? Perfection. While you can use your oven (and I will tell you how), using a decarboxylator has a few benefits. Most importantly, it ensures a more even heating process. If your oven is anything like mine and needs some serious help because it cooks everything on the left side more, then you know what I mean. With a decarboxylator, you can be sure your cannabis is being properly and evenly decarbed. It also really helps with the smell. If you use the oven to decarboxylate, guess where the smell goes? Everywhere! Love the smell or not; it gets pretty potent. The decarboxylator does let some scent escape, but nothing like an oven does. I also highly recommend that when it is done you take the machine *outside* and open it there, as the aroma will be quite strong indoors if you don't. Let the cannabis air out and cool down for a few minutes and then transfer it to an airtight container. This will help keep your house skunk-free.

What if you don't have $200 to spend on one of these handy-dandy helpers? That's okay. A cookie sheet, your oven, and about a half an hour are all it will take to decarb on your own. Begin by grinding your cannabis and spreading it out on the cookie sheet; you may use parchment paper if you'd like, but it is not necessary. Preheat your oven to 225 degrees. Place the cookie sheet in the oven and bake for 30–40 minutes. The cannabis will brown. Once it is done, seal it in an airtight container.

This decarboxylated flower is what we will be using to make some infusions that will be used (along with the flower itself) in our recipes.

Infusions

Infusing certain products with the decarboxylated flower allows for the THC to be carried in whatever base you have chosen. Ghee, butter, oils, and even alcohol can all be infused with decarboxylated flower, giving you endless possibilities for how to add cannabis to your menu.

Again, there is equipment out there to help you do this easily, and again, without smelling up your whole house. The Magic Butter Machine is less than $200 and easily infuses your base with very little work from you. You simply follow the directions, by adding your material (flower and the base you want to infuse), selecting the correct corresponding temperature button, and then … you just wait and let it do its thing. That's it. The Magic Butter Machine even has a cleaning setting. I am amazed at how well it works, and how easy it is. The unit uses a blade that finely slices the cannabis and mixes it into your base and heats to the correct preset temperatures to speed the infusion process up. But of course, infusions can be made "by hand" if spending the extra money is not an option. By-hand options will not give you as potent a final product.

Cannabutter (or Ghee)

Cannabutter is literally cannabis-infused butter. It can be made with butter or ghee but NOT margarine. Because of the slightly higher fat content of ghee, the cannabinoids are absorbed better, meaning more THC making happy little bonds with fat molecules. While ghee is more expensive than butter, you've already invested in the cannabis, so you might want to spend the extra money and compare the difference for yourself. Ghee will also change the flavor of what you make with its intensified rich buttery taste. When it comes down to it, it's once again up to your own personal taste and finances. I use both, but I do prefer ghee for certain recipes. When we get to the recipes, I will let you know which type of butter/ghee I use in each, but you can switch them anytime. Have plenty of paper towels on hand—working with butter and ghee can get messy quick.

CANNABUTTER (STOVE-TOP METHOD)

Ingredients

1 cup water
1 cup butter/ghee
7–10 grams ground decarboxylated cannabis

Utensils

Small saucepan
Wooden spoon
Candy thermometer
Cheesecloth
Glass bowl or jar you can fit a rubber band around
Rubber band

Place a small saucepan on the stove on low heat. Add the cup of water and bring to a low simmer. Add the butter and allow it to melt. The water will help keep the butter (or ghee) from burning. Pour in the ground cannabis. Stir gently.

Keep the concoction simmering at 175 degrees for 2–3 hours. Be sure to stir occasionally. If you need to, add more water to keep the butter or ghee from burning. Do not let the mixture boil. While the butter is simmering, set up your jar or bowl by covering it with cheesecloth and securing the cloth around the top of the jar or bowl with a rubber band.

Allow the butter to cool a bit, then carefully pour over the cheesecloth. There are two schools of thought about what to do next. You can either allow the cannabis to sit and drip on its own, which can take a while and won't give you the most value for your dollar, or you can wrap the cheesecloth up with the plant inside and squeeze out every last drop you can get. I'm a squeezer. Squeezing does run the risk of adding some plant material back into the butter, so again this is up to you and your own personal taste. Split your first batch in half, try it both ways, and see if it makes a noticeable difference to your taste buds or not. When it's all strained, store the butter or ghee in an airtight container in the refrigerator. Don't throw out your leftover plant material. It still has some good stuff in it that you can use in other recipes. Keep it refrigerated in an airtight container too.

CANNABUTTER (SLOW COOKER METHOD)

Ingredients

¼ cup water

1 cup butter/ghee

7–10 grams ground decarboxylated cannabis

Utensils

Slow cooker

Wooden spoon

Cheesecloth

Glass bowl or jar you can fit a rubber band around

Rubber band

Place water and butter or ghee into the slow cooker. Set temperature to 160. (You may go up to 190, but do not exceed 200 degrees.) Allow butter to melt, add cannabis, and stir. Cook for at least 3 hours. Allow to cool and strain with the same method as the previous recipe.

Using slightly higher temperatures and cook times helps speed up and maximize the infusion process. Longer with more heat will give stronger infusions, but you don't want to overdo it either. Too much heat for too long starts to break down terpenes and cannabinoids.

CANNA OILS

Cooking oils and other carrier oils can be infused with cannabis, but once again we want to look for high fat content. Unrefined coconut oil and olive oil are the two most popular to use. I use them both, depending on my recipe. Of course, canna oils don't only have to be used for cooking—they can be used to make pain relief and massage oils too.

Ingredients
1 cup oil of your choice
7–10 grams ground decarboxylated cannabis

Utensils
Double boiler or slow cooker
Wooden spoon
Items for straining

Place oil and ground cannabis in the double boiler/slow cooker and mix well with a wooden spoon. If using a double boiler, cook on low for 6–8 hours. Slow cookers can be set to low for 4–6 hours. Be sure oil temperature does not exceed 240 degrees. Allow oil to cool, then strain.

ALCOHOL INFUSIONS

This topic may be a bit touchy for some, and I completely understand why. Combining alcohol with cannabis adds a whole new elephant to the mix. But this book is about personal preferences, and how to make cannabis best work for YOU. Besides, we're all adults here and capable of making our own choices. I wouldn't recommend using it in this form often, though some medicinal patients may use tinctures daily. But having a spiritual experience with friends under a full moon might be a little more spiritual with a glass of canna-champagne laced with violets and lavender. Or perhaps a Samhain drum circle with spiced cannabis hard cider?

The best alcohol infusions are going to be done with hard alcohols. It is possible to infuse wine and champagne, as long as you have a good wine stopper for the bottle so that the cannabis has time to sit in the alcohol without it going flat. The exception to this would be if you were making a drink such as a warm mulled wine, because then you can heat it anyway. You can also make an Everclear tincture and then add drops of that into a champagne or wine. There are many ways to incorporate cannabis into cocktails, and of course mocktails as well.

While any alcohol can be infused on the stove, when it comes to Everclear (grain alcohol), I'm too chicken. Everclear is highly flammable, so I simply do not infuse it on my stove. Anything else I'm going to infuse using the stove is fine. You can also use a slow cooker if the temperature is low enough. The alcohol should never exceed 160 degrees.

Before infusing alcohol, it's important to take the amounts into effect. Everclear is made as a tincture, so the ratio between cannabis and alcohol will be close. This gives us a good strong tincture so that we only need milliliters of it instead of ounces. However, when you are infusing other hard liquors, you will need even less. With wine or champagne, you will want to use even less cannabis still. Particularly with wine and champagne, you do not want to overpower your drink with the taste of the cannabis; because you will most likely consume more at a time, you want it weaker to begin with.

For Gold Dragon (the name for an infusion made with Everclear and decarboxylated cannabis), I use 7 grams of cannabis to 1 cup of Everclear. With brandy, whiskey, rum, vodka, tequila, and other hard liquors I use 3½ grams cannabis to 6 cups alcohol. For wine and champagne, I use a ½ gram per 750 ml bottle. You are certainly free to use more once you get used to using it, or less if you find this to be too much. When I am infusing alcohol for mixed drinks and beverages, I prefer it to be a light complement. I also wouldn't drink an entire bottle of infused wine by myself. This isn't your "oh hell yeah, let's party" type of drink. The beverages we will create are for meditative, ritualistic, or other spiritual purposes. They are for small sipping pleasures, not shots.

Let's begin with the Everclear Gold Dragon infusion. You don't need to make too much of this at a time; a little will go a long way. Fill a glass jar (save one from pickles or mustard or something like that to reuse) with 1 cup of Everclear and 7 grams of decarboxylated cannabis. Replace lid tightly and shake to mix. Often you are told to store things in a cool, dark location, but not this one; keeping it in a warm area will help the process along. The longer you allow the cannabis to infuse the Everclear, the more potent your result will be. Allow it to sit for at least four weeks, giving it a shake every day. Strain before storing. For dosing, you will be needing a dropper marked with milliliters. You can also imbue your infusion with the energy of the full moon by placing it outside every month under the light of the moon.

Hard liquors can also be prepared in the same manner as the Everclear, but if you are in a hurry, these can be done on the stove or in a slow cooker in a short time. Again, I recommend 3½ grams to 6 cups, but you can make it as strong as you like, as long as you practice with it safely. Alcohol and cannabis can be gently simmered at no more than 160 degrees for 20–30 minutes. Strain to store.

Tip: If you think your infusion is too strong, you can "water" it down by adding another cup of the same alcohol.

To infuse wine or champagne, open the bottle and place a ½ gram inside. Recork, then allow the cannabis to settle. You will need to gently swirl the bottle each day. Allow it to sit for at least a week. Strain to store.

As I stated earlier, red wine can also be infused with heat if you are going to be making a warm mulled red wine. Allow the wine to simmer for 20 minutes at less than 160 degrees.

CANNA HONEY

Combining these two gifts of the goddess together is one of my favorite ways to consume cannabis in an edible form. Not only can the honey be cooked and baked with, it can be used in teas and other beverages. It's very versatile.

You can make canna honey in either a slow cooker or a Dutch oven.

You will need 3 pounds of raw organic honey, 14 grams of decarboxylated cannabis, and a cheesecloth. Tie up the cannabis in the cheesecloth. Place the cheesecloth inside the cooker and pour the honey over the top. If using a slow cooker, cook on low. If using a Dutch oven, preheat the oven to 180 degrees. Bake or slow cook for 5 hours, stirring every 20 minutes with a spatula, being sure to scrape down the sides. When done, remove the cheesecloth and squeeze out as much honey as you can. Save the honey-soaked cannabis for one of our recipes, or use it for whatever you'd prefer.

CANNA SYRUP

Simple syrup is a key ingredient in many cocktails, so infusing it with cannabis is another way to add cannabis to your beverages. This recipe is from Warren Bobrow's *Cannabis Cocktails, Mocktails & Tonics* (Bobrow 2016, 43). You will need a saucepan with a lid, and a candy thermometer.

Ingredients

2 cups filtered spring water
1 cup raw (organic) honey
4 grams finely ground decarbed cannabis
1 tablespoon vegetarian liquid lecithin

Bring water to a roaring boil in a saucepan. Reduce temperature to 190 degrees. Add raw honey and stir until it's totally dissolved. Add cannabis, cover saucepan, and reduce temp to 160 degrees. Simmer for at least 30 minutes. Reduce heat to medium-low and add the lecithin. Cook for another 10 minutes, stirring constantly. Remove from heat and strain through cheesecloth.

Recipes: Putting It into Practice

Now that we know how to infuse our base ingredients, the sky is the limit for what you can try. A recipe calls for oil? You got it! Butter? You got it! Decarboxylated flower (and leftover plant material strained from infusions) can also be chopped up and added to recipes. For some people, the taste can be an issue, so there are ways to work around that by increasing other flavorings or spices.

The recipes I am including are perfect for either a special treat for yourself or for groups practicing together.

There are other ways of cooking with cannabis, such as working with concentrates. In states where edible concentrate oil is available, this can be added to your foods as well with a lot less fuss. Since this book is directed more toward beginners, I am going to keep the cooking with cannabis skills at a beginner level. There are many great cannabis cookbooks already on the market, and with this being such a young and booming industry, there are bound to be incredible new releases all the time.

PAN'S STUFFED MUSHROOMS

Servings: approximately 24 mushrooms (depending on size)
Total creation time: 35 minutes

Ingredients

1½ cups water

2 tablespoons cannabutter

2 tablespoons butter (regular)

1 teaspoon ground sage

1 teaspoon ground and finely chopped
    decarboxylated cannabis flower

1 box or bag of stuffing (6 ounces makes
    approximately 2 dozen mushrooms)

1 pound mushroom caps, destemmed and cleaned
    (either white button or baby portabella)

Ground pepper to taste

Add water, both butters, sage, and cannabis flower to a medium-size pot on the stove. Warm water enough for butter to melt, stirring until well blended. Pour in stuffing and stir until well coated and moist all over. Fill mushrooms to overflowing and place into a casserole dish. Sprinkle with fresh ground pepper. Bake 20–25 minutes at 375 degrees.

These make a great easy-to-share appetizer. Between the butter and the flower, they pack a punch.

BAKED CHEESE SL-HIGH-DERS

Servings: 12

Total creation time: 15 minutes

Ingredients

Package of Hawaiian rolls (do not separate)

Sliced havarti (one slice will cover 4 rolls)

Sliced smoked gouda (one slice will cover 4 rolls)

2 tablespoons cannabutter, melted

Preheat oven to 325 degrees.

Grease casserole dish. Using a large bread knife, cut horizontally through all the rolls (still connected together) making a full top and a full bottom.

Put bottom half in the casserole dish. Use a pastry brush to brush melted cannabutter on the top side of the bottom half of the rolls. Cover the bottom half with cheese slices using a single layer of each type.

Place the top on and brush it with melted cannabutter.

Bake for 10 minutes, until the cheese is melted.

Easy to make a few or a bunch at once! When I first tried this out, I told my friend these would be great for when you have the munchies, and then they give you the munchies! The sweetness of the Hawaiian rolls helps offset the weed taste of the cannabutter.

BAKED BRIE

Servings: approximately 24
Total creation time: 50 minutes

Ingredients

8 sheets of phyllo dough (be sure it is fully thawed before trying to pick
 it up and separate from the roll)
4 tablespoons melted cannabutter
1 wheel of brie
1 egg, beaten

Preheat oven to 325 degrees.

Lay out a sheet of phyllo dough on a baking sheet. (Keep phyllo not being used under a damp paper towel, as it dries out very quickly.) Gently brush with melted butter. Place another sheet on top, and, again, gently brush with melted butter. You do not want to soak the sheets, so be careful with how much you use. Repeat the process until you have stacked and buttered all 8 sheets. Place the brie in the center of the dough and wrap it up by folding the dough over the top all the way around. Brush the top again with more butter, then with the beaten egg wash. Bake for 35–40 minutes. Allow to cool 10 minutes before serving with crackers.

Baked brie is incredible no matter what, so adding a hint of THC to it can only make it even more divine.

Because you will be using such a small amount of butter here, you might want to use a higher concentration cannabutter.

THE DEVIL'S EGGS

Servings: 12
Total creation time: 1 hour

Ingredients

6 hardboiled eggs
2 tablespoons oil
3 tablespoons cooked, diced bacon
1 teaspoon Dijon mustard
1 tablespoon canned green chilies, chopped
1 tablespoon diced red onion
4 tablespoons coconut canna oil

Slice the eggs in half the long way, scooping the yolks into a bowl. Put the whites on a plate. Smash yolks in a bowl with a fork. Add the rest of the ingredients and mix well. Scoop mixture back into the egg whites and chill for 30 minutes.

Yes, Pagans get flack and people think we worship the devil. Nope. Not why these are called the Devil's Eggs. It's not even for the use of "devil's weed." Not at all. It's the bacon, onion, and green chilies that gave these eggs their name. I love them!

These eggs are divine—and loaded with canna oil. Perfect for maintaining a high.

HIGH THYME MEATBALLS

Servings: approximately 12
Total creation time: 35 minutes

Ingredients

1 pound ground beef

3 tablespoons chopped onion

2 cloves garlic, minced

2 tablespoons bread crumbs

2 tablespoons grated Parmesan cheese

1 egg, beaten

1 tablespoon dried oregano

2 teaspoons dried thyme

2 tablespoons steak sauce

1 teaspoon salt

½ teaspoon white pepper

Preheat oven to 350 degrees.

Mix all ingredients together by hand in a large bowl. Roll into balls about 1½ inches in diameter. Place on a cookie sheet and bake for 15 minutes. Be sure centers are fully cooked.

Easy to make and bake. Perfect dipped in a sweet and sour sauce (if you have edible oil available to you, add a little to your sauce for more potency) or marinara. Serve with toothpicks for easy dipping.

LORD SHIVA'S SPICED NUTS

Servings: approximately 12
Total creation time: 30 minutes

Ingredients
1½ cups cashews
1½ cups pecans
1 cup Brazil nuts
1 teaspoon curry powder
1 teaspoon ground cumin
½ teaspoon ground cardamom
Sprinkle of cayenne pepper (to taste)
Sea salt
3 tablespoons coconut canna oil (you may substitute canna olive oil)

Preheat oven to 300 degrees.

Mix nuts together. Blend dry ingredients together and then add oil. Mix well. Pour over nuts, mixing as you go and ensuring they are all covered. Spread out in a single layer on a cookie sheet. Bake for 20 minutes, stirring every 5 minutes.

These Indian spiced nuts are the perfect complement for many of your meditations, particularly when calling in the Divine Masculine.

GREEN FAIRY LAVENDER COOKIES

Servings: approximately 24
Total creation time: 30 minutes

Ingredients

1 cup cannabutter
¾ cup sugar
¼ cup brown sugar
2 eggs (at room temperature)
½ teaspoon baking soda
1 teaspoon salt
4 teaspoons vanilla extract
2¼ cups flour
2 tablespoons finely ground lavender buds

Preheat oven to 325.

Use a hand mixer to blend butter, sugars, and eggs together. When smooth and well blended, add baking soda, salt, and vanilla extract and blend. Use a large spatula to blend in the flour. When everything is well blended, add lavender buds and mix well. Scoop balls with a tablespoon and place on a baking sheet. Bake for 8–10 minutes. Keep a close eye on them to ensure they bake all the way through but don't burn.

The light, peaceful combination of lavender and vanilla is both aromatic and relaxing. The effect of these cookies is purely magical.

SALTED CARAMEL OOEY GOOEY CHOCOLATY BARS OF GOODNESS

Servings: approximately 12

Total creation time: 1 hour, 15 minutes

Ingredients

2 cups sugar

1 cup baking cocoa

1 cup canna coconut oil

½ cup milk

¼ cup RumChata

4 eggs

1 teaspoon salt

1 teaspoon baking powder

1½ cups flour

1 10-ounce bag mini chocolate chips

11 ounces caramel baking candy

11 ounces sweetened condensed milk

1 tablespoon course sea salt or pink Himalayan salt

Preheat oven to 350 degrees.

Grease a 9 x 13-inch pan. Using a hand mixer, combine the sugar, cocoa, oil, milk, RumChata, and egg. Blend well. Add salt and baking powder to the mixture and blend. Slowly add flour, blending it in as you go. Switch to a large spatula and mix in the mini chips.

Spread a little more than half of the mixture into the bottom of the pan, smoothing it out all over. The mix will be very thick. Bake for 14 minutes.

While that layer bakes, place the caramel in a glass bowl and microwave for 30 seconds. Add the sweetened condensed milk and heat for another 30 seconds. Stir as much as you can and then heat for another 30 seconds. You will need to do this 3–4 times until the caramel blends completely with the milk.

After the 14 minutes have passed, remove the pan from the oven and slowly pour caramel mixture all over the top. Sprinkle the salt all over the caramel. Because the brownie mixture is so thick, the second layer must be "plopped" down to avoid having to spread it as much as possible. Use a tablespoon to plop batter blobs down close enough to touch each other. Gently spread batter where needed to cover as well as you can.

Bake for another 40–45 minutes. Check center with a toothpick to see if it is done.

These are basically highly caramel-infused brownies. They are RICH. A little goes a long way because they are so decadent and high in THC.

ZEN GARDEN FRUIT DELIGHT

Servings: 8
Total creation time: at least 30 minutes

Ingredients
1 cup citrus rum
1 cup banana rum
1 gram decarboxylated cannabis
1 tablespoon organic raw honey
1 pint strawberries
1 pint blueberries
2 cups pineapple chunks
2 cups watermelon chunks

Combine the rums in a pan on the stove and infuse with cannabis. You can do this either by tying up the cannabis in cheesecloth and soaking it in the rum, or allowing it to float freely and strain later. Heat rum on low; do not let it boil. Allow cannabis at least 20 minutes to steep. The longer you allow the cannabis to steep, the more concentrated it will be. Remove cannabis from rum. While still warm, add a tablespoon of organic raw honey. Place fruit in a bowl, pour rum over the top, and chill overnight.

In the morning, pour off the alcohol (reserving the rum if you want) and serve the fruits with toothpicks. You can make drinks with the reserved rum.

I literally came up with this by looking at what was almost empty in my liquor cabinet. I may have to do that more often because this worked out fantastically. Not only do you get infused fruit, but you can use the rum to make an awesome punch too.

PEANUT BUDDHA BALLS

Servings: approximately 24
Total creation time: 3 hours

Ingredients

1 cup peanut butter

6 tablespoons softened cannabutter

2 cups powdered sugar

16 ounces milk chocolate for melting

Using a hand mixer, combine the peanut butter and cannabutter until well blended. Slowly add some powdered sugar and mix in with a wooden spoon. Continue adding powdered sugar and blending. Do not overmix. Peanut butter should appear flat, not shiny and oily. Roll the mixture into balls an inch in diameter and refrigerate for 2 hours. When hardened, melt chocolate and dip each ball in it, covering them. Use a fork to lift them out, gently shake off the excess chocolate, and set them on wax paper for the chocolate to harden. Store in the refrigerator.

It's chocolate! It's peanut butter! It's cannabis!

These are rich, rich, rich, rich, and you will want to eat several. Just remember, they are loaded with cannabutter!

CERRIDWEN'S CIDER

Servings: 4
Total creation time: 30 minutes

Ingredients

4 cups apple cider
1 cup fresh cranberries
1 large navel orange, sliced into rings
⅛ teaspoon ground clove
⅛ teaspoon ground ginger
⅛ teaspoon ground nutmeg
¼ teaspoon ground cinnamon
1 tablespoon canna honey
1 teaspoon decarboxylated cannabis in a tea infuser ball (You can also
    use the cannabis that you used to make your canna honey.)

Place all ingredients in a pot and bring to a boil. Set temp to low and gently simmer while covered for 20 minutes. Remove from heat. Serve in mugs with some of the orange slices and cranberries in each mug.

Make this alcoholic by adding in infused whisky or infused cinnamon whisky.

This is a bold, tart, warming drink perfect for any workings that deal with gaining wisdom, or just something to drink on a cool fall or winter night.

VIN DU JARDIN

Servings: 4

Total creation time: 5 minute prep, minimum 24 hours chilling

Ingredients

1 bottle rosé wine

1 gram decarboxylated cannabis

2 tablespoons food grade lavender buds

An infusion pitcher or pitcher with cheesecloth

If you have an infusion pitcher, simply place all the ingredients where they need to go. If you do not have an infusion pitcher, tie the cannabis and lavender up in the cheesecloth, place it in a regular pitcher or carafe, and pour the wine over it. Allow it to set and chill for at least 24 hours.

This drink gives you the light taste of lavender with a little THC kick. It's perfect for spring or hot summer nights. It is uplifting and cheery and relaxing, all at the same time.

AMBROSIA SMOOTHIE

Servings: 2
Total creation time: 5 minutes

Ingredients

1 cup watermelon, cut into chunks

2 cups blueberries

1 cup pomegranate juice

1 tablespoon honey (this can be canna honey if you want to boost the THC level)

2 tablespoons canna oil (while I prefer the taste of coconut oil in this, it is more difficult to blend with the other items)

2 cups ice

Put everything but the ice in a blender and puree. Once it is well-blended, add the ice and puree again.

Cannabis is a healthier alternative to many medicines, and you can make healthy foods with it too. This smoothie is nectar for the gods—sweet, natural, and yummy!

CUCHULAINN'S MEDITATION TEA

Servings: 1
Total creation time: 15 minutes

Ingredients
Food grade lavender flower buds
Food grade chamomile flowers
Decarboxylated cannabis
Canna honey to taste

For each cup of tea, use 1 tablespoon of lavender, 1 tablespoon of chamomile, and ¼ teaspoon cannabis.

If you are making this for your solitary practice, you should still make a couple of cups at a time; refrigerate any tea you don't use.

Tie the lavender and cannabis up in cheesecloth and add to a pot of hot water on the stove. Keep it just below a low simmer for 10 minutes.

You can also make large batches of this using the low setting on a slow cooker. The longer you let it set, the stronger it will be both in flavor and potency.

This is my new favorite tea. It's smooth, it's relaxing, it's downright groovy, and enough of it will help you sleep at night.

MELLOW MERLOT

Servings: 4
Total creation time: at least 3 hours

Ingredients

2 cinnamon sticks
2 whole cloves
2 whole allspice
1 gram decarboxylated cannabis
1 bottle merlot
1 cup apple juice

Tie spices and cannabis up in a cheesecloth. Pour merlot and apple juice into a crockpot, then add the spice bundle. Set on low–medium for several hours. The longer you leave it, the stronger it will be both in flavor and THC content.

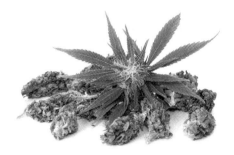

Conclusion

Writing this book was such an incredible pleasure for me. Cannabis has changed my life in so many ways. While I will not say it is a cure-all, I will say it is a truly amazing plant that, sadly, has been demonized in the United States, therefore leaving millions of people unable to reap its benefits. As more people become educated about the history and true effects of cannabis and the tide turns, more and more people are able to learn about this remarkable plant and see how it can help them in their own lives. We must not stay silent about the discrimination this plant and its users have been subjected to, but instead must open our eyes to see the truth, our minds to experience the truth, and our mouths to share the truth.

You can join me at the Wake, Bake & Meditate Facebook group and Wake, Bake & Meditate YouTube channel. I am also available at the @AuthorKerriConnor or @TheWeedWitchAuthor Facebook pages. These are places you will be able to go for support, camaraderie, and fellowship.

Journeys can be difficult, no matter how much we want to take them. I wish you success and happiness as you set out on yours.

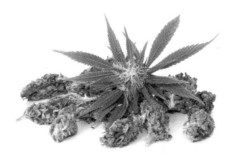

Appendix I
Possible Side Effects of Cannabis Use

- Red, itchy, or dry eyes
- Dry "cotton" mouth
- Increased blood pressure
- Increased heart rate
- Slower reaction time
- Distorted sensory perception
- Short-term memory loss
- Loss of motor skills
- Impaired mental/cognitive functioning

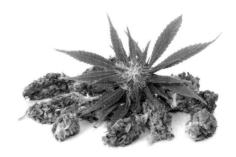

Appendix II
If You Consume Too Much

Here are some tips for dealing with intense side effects:

- Do your deep breathing exercise on a five-count cycle (inhale for five, hold for five, exhale for five).
- Remind yourself that panic is temporary. You are okay.
- Drink fruit juice or something sugary to increase your blood sugar, bringing you to a calmer state of mind and body. Be sure not to consume any energy drinks.
- CBD and limonene counteract the effects of THC. Consume some CBD and eat an orange.
- Inhale lemon essential oil.
- Lie on your side.

- Close your eyes and relax. Can you turn the experience around? Look for your safe place, but know that it is okay if you can't find it.
- If you are working with a partner, know that your partner will be there to help you through. This is what they are there for.

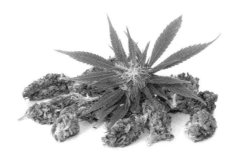

Recommended Reading

"Marijuana and the Body-Mind" by Joan Bello, in *Cannabis and Spirituality: An Explorer's Guide to an Ancient Plant Spirit Ally* by Stephen Gray.

"The Endocannabinoid System" by Gregory L. Gerdeman PhD and Jason B. Schechter PhD, in *The Pot Book: A Complete Guide to Cannabis: Its Role in Medicine, Politics, Science, and Culture* edited by Julie Holland.

"Here Are 10 Types of Marijuana That Will Make You More Spiritual" by Kent Gruetzmacher on *The Fresh Toast*.

The Cannabis Kitchen Cookbook: Feel-Good Food for Home Cooks by Robyn Griggs Lawrence and Jane West.

The Leafly Guide to Cannabis: A Handbook for the Modern Consumer by Leafly Team.

"The Best Cannabis Strains for Meditation" by Bailey Rahn on *Leafly*.

"Top 5 Strains for Yoga and Meditation" by Dana Smith on *Cannabis.net*.

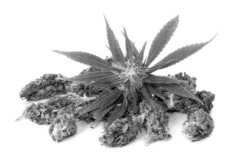

Bibliography

Bennett, Chris. "Venerable Traditions: A Brief History of the Ritual and Religious Use of Cannabis." In *Cannabis and Spirituality: An Explorer's Guide to an Ancient Plant Spirit Ally*, edited by Stephen Gray, 38–58. Rochester, VT: Park Street Press, 2017.

Bobrow, Warren. *Cannabis Cocktails, Mocktails & Tonics: The Art of Spirited Drinks and Buzz-Worthy Libations*. Beverly, MA: Fair Winds Press, 2016.

Dussault, Dee. *Ganja Yoga: A Practical Guide to Conscious Relaxation, Soothing Pain Relief, and Enlightened Self-Discovery*. San Francisco: HarperOne, 2017.

Ferrara, Mark S. *Sacred Bliss: A Spiritual History of Cannabis*. Lanham, MD: Rowman and Littlefield Publishing Group, 2016.

Gray, Stephen, ed. *Cannabis and Spirituality: An Explorer's Guide to an Ancient Plant Spirit Ally*. Rochester, VT: Park Street Press, 2017.

Harrison, Kathleen. "Who Is She? The Personification of Cannabis in Cultural and Individual Experience." In *Cannabis and Spirituality: An Explorer's Guide to an Ancient Plant Spirit Ally*, edited by Stephen Gray, 18–37. Rochester, VT: Park Street Press, 2017.

To Write to the Author

If you wish to contact the author or would like more information about this book, please write to the author in care of Llewellyn Worldwide Ltd. and we will forward your request. Both the author and publisher appreciate hearing from you and learning of your enjoyment of this book and how it has helped you. Llewellyn Worldwide Ltd. cannot guarantee that every letter written to the author can be answered, but all will be forwarded. Please write to:

Kerri Connor
℅ Llewellyn Worldwide
2143 Wooddale Drive
Woodbury, MN 55125-2989
Please enclose a self-addressed stamped envelope for reply,
or $1.00 to cover costs. If outside the U.S.A., enclose
an international postal reply coupon.

Many of Llewellyn's authors have websites with additional information and resources. For more information, please visit our website at http://www.llewellyn.com.